Abnormal Pap Smears

Abnormal Pap Smears

What Every Woman Needs to Know

Lynda Rushing, M.D., and Nancy Joste, M.D.

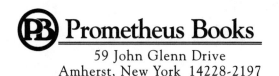

Prometheus Books

59 John Glenn Drive
Amherst, New York 14228-2197

Illustrations by Thomas J. Gagliano, Gagliano Graphics

Published 2001 by Prometheus Books

Inquiries should be addressed to
Prometheus Books
59 John Glenn Drive
Amherst, New York 14228–2197
VOICE: 716–691–0133, ext. 207
FAX: 716–564–2711
WWW.PROMETHEUSBOOKS.COM

05 04 03 02 01   5 4 3 2

Library of Congress Cataloging-in-Publication Data

Rushing, Lynda, 1957–
    Abnormal pap smears : What every woman needs to know / Lynda Rushing and Nancy Joste ; forewords by Christopher P. Crum and Stephen A. Cannistra.
        p. cm.
    Includes bibliographical references and index.
    ISBN 1–57392–929–8 (pbk. : alk. paper)
    1. Pap test. 2. Cervix uteri—Cancer—Diagnosis. 3. Cervix uteri—Cancer—Prevention. 4. Women—Diseases—Prevention. 5. Consumer education. I. Joste, Nancy, 1955– II. Title.

RG107.5.P3 R87 2001
616.99'466—dc21   2001031619

Printed in the United States of America on acid-free paper

To the memories of

Dr. Ramzi S. Cotran, chairman of the Department of Pathology,
Brigham and Women's Hospital (1974–2000)

and

Mary Silcox Joste

Contents

Foreword

CHRISTOPHER P. CRUM, M.D.

Out of every two hundred women, three will develop cervical cancer and one will die of this disease. This should not happen. A simple speculum exam can place the cervix in plain sight, and accessible to a time-honored foundation of cancer prevention, the Papanicolaou smear. Abnormal cells are shed from the cervix months to years prior to the onset of cancer and their detection and early treatment will both preserve fertility and reduce the risk of cancer to fewer than one in 500. Overall, cancer rates have fallen by over two-thirds since the introduction of the Papanicolaou smear fifty years ago.

But as a potentially preventable disease, cervical cancer is at once both tantalizing and exasperating. Nearly fifteen thousand women still contract cervical cancer every year in the United States and nearly five thousand will die of the disease. In a culture with the highest standard of living and most comprehensive and costly health care in the world, at least one-half of cervical cancer victims have not had regular Papanicolaou smears. The remainder did, but were victims of inevitable deficiencies in the system. The Pap smear may have missed the abnormal cells. The cytopathologist may have missed the cells when examining the smear; the physician may not have appreciated the significance of the smear abnormality or counsel the patient of her risks; the patient may have ignored the warnings of her physician, or she may have simply been an unlucky victim of a cancer that could not be prevented in the context of reasonable care.

We examine millions of women with abnormal Pap smears every year.

Ask any woman, and more often than not she will be able to describe this ordeal. But she will not have cancer. So how is the medical profession going to find those fifteen thousand women destined for cancer every year and rescue them? Should we require that every woman have a Papanicolaou smear? Should we test every woman for human papillomavirus, a necessary ingredient in cancer development but also a ubiquitous infection? Should we examine the cervix of every woman every year? What will it take to eliminate cervical cancer?

The answer rests with you. You can read this book in an afternoon. In it two highly respected women physicians will escort you through the maze of cervical cancer prevention. You will gain knowledge that will empower you to control your fear of this disease and place the abnormal Pap smear and its causes in perspective. For some of you, this book is a wake-up call to get your first Papanicolaou smear. For others, it is an insurance policy against ignorance, embarrassment, and fear. For the few of you destined to join the fifteen thousand women with cervical cancer this year or the next, this book could reverse your fortunes. It could very well save your life.

Christopher P. Crum, M.D.
Professor of Pathology, Harvard Medical School
Director, Women's and Perinatal Pathology
Brigham and Women's Hospital
Boston, Massachusetts

Foreword

STEPHEN A. CANNISTRA, M.D.

Drs. Lynda Rushing and Nancy Joste have written a valuable book designed to empower women by providing much needed knowledge about cervical screening and diagnosis through the use of the Pap smear test. From the patient's point of view, such tests are shrouded in mystery, which can lead to considerable and unnecessary anxiety. This book succeeds in clarifying many of the issues women face after being told that their Pap smear is "abnormal." Readers will find many useful questions raised in each chapter, questions that address the most common concerns raised by patients as they receive their test results, discuss the likely diagnosis, and, if necessary, choose from possible treatment options. Importantly, chapters devoted to understanding the diagnostic process and describing individual experiences offer a unique opportunity for women to gain insight into their own bodies at a personal level. There is therapeutic value to knowing that others have experienced the same fears and have overcome their anxiety. In many ways, cervical screening represents a success story of modern medicine, and this book makes the point clear in a way that patients and their families can understand and appreciate.

Obviously, no book can replace the good medical advice one can obtain from discussing health concerns directly with a qualified physician. The purpose of this helpful work is not to make treatment recommendations, but to serve as a tool for women to ask the right questions, gain a better understanding of the recommendations made by their physicians, and work with their gynecologists to make decisions that are right for their particular situations. This book achieves these goals very well and should be an excellent resource for patients and their families.

Stephen A. Cannistra, M.D.
Associate Professor of Medicine, Harvard Medical School
Director, Gynecologic Medical Oncology
Beth Israel Deaconess Medical Center
Boston, Massachusetts

Preface

The idea for this book came about during a telephone conversation we had a few years ago when we learned that we were having similar experiences as medical directors of cytology laboratories. It seemed that wherever we went, we ran into women with abnormal Pap smear diagnoses who wanted to discuss them. We are both cytopathologists having spent years training for our professions and then most of our working days thereafter diagnosing abnormal Pap smears. We were flabbergasted to discover that not many women even knew what our diagnoses meant. Beyond understanding that they had an abnormal Pap smear, most women we spoke with did not know the probable causes of abnormal cells on that test or even that the Pap smear looked for effects of an infection, that of the human papillomavirus (HPV). Further, almost no one understood that this virus is sexually transmitted and is also the causative agent of cervical cancer. To say that we were naïve is an understatement. We felt strongly the need for a guide such as this one to help women navigate the often murky waters of cervical disease. We became committed to producing such a guide, in language that was clear and as free as possible from confusing medical jargon.

As we delved deeper into this process, however, we began to realize that the need for this information was urgent. Although human papillomavirus is thought to be the most common sexually transmitted infection, we were shocked to hear women with this infection, particularly young women, talk about the guilt and shame they felt when they discovered that their cervical problems were related to HPV. Some women isolated themselves, not talking

13

to friends or family for fear that they would appear promiscuous. They dealt with this infection alone and in fear. One teenager went to great pains to shield this information from her (first) boyfriend, when clearly he was the source of her infection!

Other women did not know what to expect in the course of their workups for abnormal Pap smears and were distressed at the invasive and frequently painful nature of some of their follow-up tests. One woman became hysterical when she heard the word "biopsy." She explained to us—the uncomprehending physicians—that the word was fraught with scary imagery for the average nonmedical person. Another woman, who considered herself to be quite modest, was deeply upset every time she had to undergo a closer visualization of her cervix, normally a painless procedure.

We spoke with several brave women who were diagnosed with cervical cancer. One such woman had never had a Pap smear in her life and feared for the lives of her daughters, none of whom she could convince to have Pap smears. We joined her in her feelings of helplessness as we gazed at pictures of her six beautiful daughters.

We also spoke to women who gave us hope. These were women who had close and supportive relationships with their healthcare providers. They actively sought to both educate themselves on their cervical conditions and educate the clinicians on their needs as patients.

Our goal in writing this book is a similar one: we want to familiarize as many women as possible about the significance of an abnormal Pap smear and its relationship to human papillomavirus and cervical cancer. We want to encourage all women to open a dialog with their clinicians so that health professionals can help them understand the odds for developing cervical cancer and in so doing help women everywhere to beat the odds. We will be presenting some of this information in the context of stories from other women who have received abnormal or unclear Pap smear results—this in the hope that their experiences and suggestions can help others.

We are also committed to publicizing the widespread nature of human papillomaviruses and their association with cervical cancer. As physicians and as mothers of young daughters, we want to help teach our young women who are sexually active to take care of their bodies and to educate themselves about the consequences of their behavior. We hope this information will serve to reduce the preventable tragedy of cervical cancer in this country and throughout the world.

Acknowledgments

We would like to thank the following individuals for their invaluable assistance and helpful comments on portions of this book:

In Boston: Dr. Christopher Crum, professor of pathology, Harvard Medical School and director, Gynecologic and Perinatal Pathology, Brigham and Women's Hospital; Dr. Anthony DiSciullo, assistant clinical professor of Obstetrics, Gynecology, and Reproductive Biology, Harvard Medical School and director of the Division of Gynecology, Mount Auburn Hospital; Dr. Young Kim, assistant professor of Obstetrics, Gynecology, and Reproductive Biology, Harvard Medical School and staff gynecologic oncologist, Beth Israel Deaconess Hospital; Dr. Diane McGrory, staff gynecologist, Newton-Wellesley Hospital; and Ms. Bronya Bellerose, supervisor, Pathology Services, Inc.

In Albuquerque: All at the University of New Mexico Health Sciences Center School of Medicine—Dr. Cosette Wheeler, associate professor, Department of Molecular Genetics and Microbiology; Dr. Harriet Smith, associate professor, Department of Obstetrics and Gynecology and director of Gynecologic Oncology; Dr. Eve Espey, assistant professor, Department of Obstetrics and Gynecology; and Dr. Meggan Zsemlye, assistant professor, Department of Obstetrics and Gynecology.

A number of individuals were invaluable in both the conception and the actual realization of this book. First of all, I would like to thank my col-

15

leagues, Dr. Imad Nasser and Dr. Kenneth Lee, for helping me with work coverage so that this project could get done. My former boss, Dr. Karl Sorger, and my current boss, Dr. Karl Proppe, were also greatly supportive of this project. I owe a debt of thanks to Dr. Christopher Crum, who has helped me immeasurably with this book as well as with my career in pathology. Thanks also to Michael Scheumeister, who helped me to stay mentally and physically strong during the often hectic course of this endeavor. My parents, James Alton Rushing and Teruko Suda Rushing, continue to be my biggest supporters. I owe them more than I could ever repay. I also have had the good fortune of coming home each night to my small but loud cheering section: my husband, Dr. Josef Gendlerman, and my two athlete-scholars, Kira Rushing Gendlerman and Emma Rushing Gendlerman. They make everything fun. Lastly, I would like to thank our editors, Mary A. Read and Steven L. Mitchell, and project manager, Christine Kramer, for their belief in this project and their always polite manner. It was much appreciated.

Lynda Rushing, M.D.

I have greatly appreciated the support of my chair, Dr. Mary Lipscomb, Department of Pathology, University of New Mexico School of Medicine. My colleagues in surgical pathology, Dr. Richard Feddersen, Dr. Thèrése Bocklage, and Dr. Marcia Wills, provided the schedule flexibility allowing me time to write this book. My family was a continuous and enthusiastic source of support: my husband, John Pietz, and my irrepressible children, Harlan and Anna Pietz. Mary A. Read at Prometheus Books never failed to provide prompt and kind advice. I am also grateful to our editor, Mr. Steven L. Mitchell, for opening the door of opportunity with publishing this book.

Nancy Joste, M.D.

O N E

Cervical Cancer and Human Papillomaviruses

SEXUALLY TRANSMITTED DISEASES

Karen, a thirty-three-year-old married mother of two, was understandably concerned when she got the call from her gynecologist's office informing her of her abnormal Pap smear, the test which checks for cervical cancer. She was a weekend athlete, in great shape, a nonsmoker who took good care of herself. She never missed a physical, was up-to-date on her mammograms, and was religious about her yearly Pap smears, which had always been normal. There was no history of cancer on either side of her family and she had no health problems. But she knew that the Pap smear was a test for cervical cancer, a disease that could strike anyone. She approached her follow-up appointment with apprehension. However, as she sat in the exam room in her thin paper gown talking to the physician's assistant, her feelings of foreboding gradually changed to confusion and finally gave way to frustration as she struggled to understand the battery of questions that was thrown at her. Had she ever had an abnormal Pap smear? Was she sure? Even in college? Was she still married to the same person or was she now seeing someone else? Did she want to be tested for other sexually transmitted diseases? Karen became alarmed. *Wasn't the Pap smear a test for cancer? What did screening for cancer have to do with sexually transmitted diseases?*

CERVICAL CANCER AND ITS PRECURSORS
APPEAR TO BE SEXUALLY TRANSMITTED

Over the last twenty-five years, extensive research has looked into the causes of cervical cancer and although much remains uncertain, one fact has become undeniable: cervical cancer behaves very much like a sexually transmitted disease. Early on, researchers noted an interesting correlation: women who have never had any sexual contact, such as nuns, do not get the disease and conversely, women who have had many male sexual partners have the highest risk of contracting cervical cancer or one of its precursors.

Cervical cancer, like many other cancers, appears to evolve through "steps" so that the earliest stage is not actually cancer but a "precancer" which has not become technically cancer since it cannot invade and destroy normal body tissues at this point. This quality of being able to invade and destroy tissues pretty much defines malignancy. As far as the cervix is concerned, there are several terms that refer to this precancerous stage. The terms "precancer," "precursor," "dysplasia," and "squamous intraepithelial lesion" or SIL are synonymous and all refer to the earliest changes that occur in cervical tissue prior to its transformation into cancer. We will usually refer to these precancerous changes as a squamous intraepithelial lesion or SIL in this book since that is what they generally are called in Pap smear reports. In chapter 3 you will see clear illustrations of SIL and cervical cancer. For now, let us focus on some early cervical cancer research.

In the United States, the peak age for developing cervical cancer precursors is among women in their twenties, which is also the peak age of sexual activity. Curiously, the peak age for developing cervical cancer is some ten to fifteen years later. Thus the disease seems to have a long "latency" or quiet period between the time of early precancer development and the time of development of a clearly malignant disease. These idiosyncrasies of cervical cancer did not escape investigators. According to medical historians as summarized by Griffiths in a 1991 article, even in the 1800s, it was thought that cervical cancer was somehow related to a sexually transmitted infection which could remain quietly in the body for many years before causing a tumor. More recently, some thought that a sexually transmitted virus was the prime suspect, but which one?

In the early to mid-1970s, cervical cancer researchers at Emory and Johns Hopkins Universities, among others, thought that a good candidate might be the herpes simplex virus. Herpes causes painful sores in and around the genital tract and was clearly related to sexual activity. Reports from these researchers suggested that this virus could be isolated from cells taken from cervical cancer. Those early studies, while valid, did not directly connect the herpes virus to cervical cancer and were quickly overtaken by reports from other researchers working with a different virus which infects the human genital tract: the human papillomavirus.

THE HUMAN PAPILLOMAVIRUS

The human papillomaviruses (or HPV) represents a family of viruses of which currently over one hundred different subtypes have been identified. These viruses are already familiar to many of us since this is the same virus group that causes the common skin warts seen on the hands and feet. HPV is a small virus characterized by having two strands of genetic material or DNA within a spherical protein shell. This virus looks somewhat like a golf ball under high magnification.

Out of the more than one hundred viral subtypes, there are a number (over forty) of HPV types that prefer to infect the human genital tract. Once passed to an individual through sexual contact, the virus makes itself at home in the cells lining a man's penis or a woman's vulva, vagina, or cervix. The virus is easily spread from person to person through the mixing of bodily fluids which occurs during sexual contact. This includes skin to skin contact, vaginal sex, anal sex, and, rarely, oral sex.

Not surprisingly, the virus can cause fleshy genital warts (or condylomas) found on the external genitals or anal areas of both men and women. Although these warts can be both embarrassing and highly contagious, they rarely lead to the development of cancer. The more dangerous HPV lesions are the subtle and difficult to see "flat" lesions that can occur on a cervix, vagina, and vulva and, less commonly, on a penis. Unlike visible genital warts, these produce no symptoms. The lesions in the cervix are the cervical cancer precursors also known as squamous intraepithelial lesions (SILs) or dysplasia. The less common vaginal lesions are known as "vaginal intraepithelial neoplasia" or VAINs and the vulvar lesions as "vulvar intraepithelial neoplasia" or VINs.

The existence of these genital viruses is not a modern phenomenon.

Their presence and association with sexual contact was observed even during the Roman era when it was noted that genital warts were a sign of previous sexual activity. However, it was only during modern times that the existence of additional papillomaviruses other than those which cause genital warts was discovered and the association of those papillomaviruses and cervical cancer was established.

CERTAIN HPVs ARE
ASSOCIATED WITH CERVICAL CANCER

In the early 1980s, a critical event for the study of cervical cancer took place when the human papillomavirus was successfully cloned (its exact genetic makeup was replicated). This event made it possible to experimentally identify HPV genetic material (DNA) in cervical cancers and their precursors as well as in genital warts. HPV genetic material was found in over 90 percent of these lesions. With current, more sensitive, techniques, this number is very close to 100 percent. Knowledge of the sexually transmitted nature of HPV and its associations with cervical cancer permitted linkage of HPV infection and cervical malignancy. With this new molecular information, the connection was now firmly established between HPV and cervical cancer. HPV was the likely cause of cervical cancer.

With research on HPV progressing at breakneck speed, attention turned to the various viral subtypes and their relationships to cervical cancer. It soon became clear that while all the forty-plus genital subtypes could be found in the cancer precursors, only specific types of HPV routinely could be isolated from actual cervical cancer cells. These subtypes have become known as "high-risk" subtypes to indicate their common association with cervical cancer. Other subtypes are known as "low-risk" since they are not associated with cancer. The most commonly seen high-risk subtypes are viral subtypes 16 and 18. Subtypes 31 and 33 are also seen in association with cervical cancer. Low-risk subtypes include subtypes 6 and 11, which are most commonly seen in genital warts and rarely, if ever, appear in cancer tissue. Infection by these two groups of HPV, high-risk and low-risk types, may result in two different, although related, types of cervical lesions. These lesions are abnormalities in the cervical tissue which can sometimes be seen by the naked eye and hence can be detected by your gynecologist. However, they very often are invisible to the examining eye and must be diagnosed using a microscope to look at cervical tissue from either a Pap smear which only samples cells or from a surgical sample of the cervix called a "cervical biopsy."

The high-risk viruses typically produce a lesion called "high-grade squamous intraepithelial lesion" (HSIL). These lesions have the greatest chance of subsequently developing into cancer. The low-risk types are most often associated with low-grade squamous intraepithelial lesions (LSIL). However, as with all of life, the situation is not always so clear-cut and, unfortunately, a substantial percentage of LSILs harbor the high-risk viruses making their biological outcome a little uncertain. In some studies, this occurs at a frequency of 80 percent although the true figure is probably somewhat lower. Clearly, many "high-risk" HPV infections do not progress to high-grade precursors or cancer.

Because of the widespread use of the Pap smear in this country, cervical cancer has become a rare disease. Actually, only a minority of women will experience an abnormal Pap smear due to a SIL. Because of this, some women might think that HPV is a rare sexually transmitted disease and that few will ever be infected with HPV in their lifetimes. While this reasoning might hold true with other infections, in the case of HPV, this view would be mistaken. Amazingly, *most women who are sexually active will develop a genital infection with HPV at some point during their lives, typically during their teens and twenties.*

HPV IS THE MOST COMMON
SEXUALLY TRANSMITTED INFECTION

While various studies disagree on the exact *prevalence* (or occurrence) of the human papillomavirus, it is clear that this virus is highly transmittable or infectious. In fact, according to Dr. Christopher Crum, professor of pathology at Harvard Medical School and an expert on HPV infections in cervical disease, *probably close to 80 percent of sexually active young women will at one time be infected by HPV and at any given moment, around 45 percent of young, sexually active American women are infected by the virus.* This works out to an estimated ten million American women with active HPV infections.

These are astonishing statistics. In other words, by being a sexually active woman in the United States in the twenty-first century, the likelihood of becoming infected by HPV, the cause of cervical cancer, is almost inescapable. Contrast this to the chances of contracting a gonorrheal infection, which is less than 1 percent.

So, are the majority of American women in imminent danger of developing cervical cancer? Thankfully, the answer is no. Actually, only a small percentage of all women who develop an HPV infection go on to develop cervical lesions (about one million women) and only a small percentage of those women will develop cancer of the cervix years later (figure 1-1). This is because of an odd tendency of HPV, namely, its capacity to "regress" or disappear.

HPV: THE DISAPPEARING VIRUS

Researchers in Finland were among the first to write about an interesting feature of low-grade SILs that had been noticed by others around the world. Namely, very often these lesions seem to disappear without a trace and women in this category did not appear to have any further problems with HPV-related lesions or Pap smear abnormalities. With further studies using molecular biology techniques, it became clear that HPV infections with low-risk viral subtypes in general had a high regression rate. In other words, while many women become infected with the virus, a large majority (around 60 percent) of those women somehow "cleared" the virus from their bodies. Although it is likely that this viral clearance must involve a woman's immune system in some way, just precisely how it happens remains unknown. Suffice it to say that this virus-clearing mechanism in most women prevents an HPV infection from always resulting in a full-blown squamous intraepithelial lesion.

Our knowledge of the course of genital HPV infections is still evolving and much remains unclear. We are, however, beginning to understand the natural history of this virus. It appears that HPV infections in most women is a short-lived infection that produces no precancerous lesions. After initial exposure during sex, it takes somewhere between 6 weeks and 6 months for the virus to be detected in a woman. For most women, the virus is no longer detectable in 12 to 18 months.

For a small number of women, the virus will not disappear but will remain present in a persistent infection with no outward symptoms. These women are at risk for precancers. In some of these women, HPV may cause

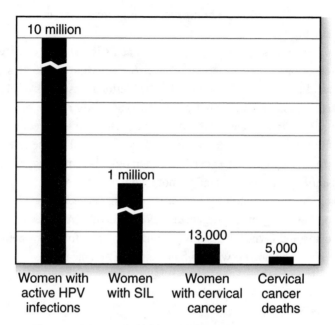

Figure 1-1. Human papillomavirus (HPV) infection and
HPV-related cervical diseases in the United States.

a SIL to form in a relatively short period of time. For other women, this process may take years. A SIL, whether appearing sooner or later, may itself persist or disappear. There is currently no way to predict the outcome of an HPV infection in a woman.

Although the human body is capable of clearing "high-risk" viruses from a woman's genital tract, they are less likely to do so. This is unfortunate, since you'll remember that these viral subtypes are more likely to lead to high-grade cancer precursors and then on to cervical cancer than are the low-risk viruses. It is estimated that fewer than 30 percent of the HSILs will regress on their own and somewhere between 11 percent and 35 percent will progress to cancer if left untreated.

The body's own natural healing of an HPV lesion via its immune system is certainly a convenient (and cheap!) way for a woman to get rid of her pre-cancer, however it obviously cannot be relied upon. A number of successful treatments are currently available to those with precancerous lesions. This topic will be discussed in chapter 4. It is clearly critical for women to have regular gynecologic health care including Pap smears so that any HPV lesion which arises may be detected and successfully treated at an early "precancerous" stage.

How often women should receive Pap smears is a subject of debate. The recommendations of the American Cancer Society and the Centers for Disease Control that are also supported by the National Institutes of Health are for annual Pap smears in sexually active women. After three or more consecutive normal Pap smears, the test may be performed less frequently at the discretion of the physician. However, studies conducted by the International Agency for Research on Cancer and other organizations suggest that less than annual Pap smears will lead to more women with cervical cancer which could have been prevented by annual Pap tests. These findings have led to recommendations by many organizations such as the American College of Obstetricians and Gynecologists for annual Pap tests for all women. In this book we also recommend women have annual Pap smears.

WHAT IS KNOWN ABOUT CERVICAL CANCER RISK FACTORS?

Over the years, certain risk factors have been identified for cervical cancer. Not surprisingly, there is a strong correlation between a woman's sexual history and her chances of developing cervical cancer. Researchers at the National Cancer Institute in the 1980s noted that women who were at a young age (before the age of sixteen) when they first had sexual intercourse are at an even higher risk for cervical cancer. It is thought that the maturing female cervix at puberty is particularly susceptible to HPV infection and is more vulnerable to tumor-producing influences. Women with multiple sexual partners and women with a male partner who has had multiple sexual partners are also at greater risk for cervical cancer. As you might imagine, this also increases the risk to teenagers since the earlier a teen becomes sexually active, the more lifetime sexual partners she is likely to have.

Other, less important potential risk factors have been identified, all of which are not well understood in the way they contribute to cervical cancer risk. These include cigarette smoking, use of oral contraceptives, infection by other sexually transmitted diseases, low socioeconomic status, race, having multiple children, and a family history of cervical cancer.

As we have noted previously, the vast majority of sexually active women have been exposed to HPV at one time or another, but only a small fraction of them will develop precancers. Clearly factors other than just HPV infection are at play in the development of SILs and cervical cancer. Medical scientists believe that a critical factor in a woman's development of cervical cancer is the ability of her own immune system to successfully counter an HPV infection. Immunosuppression in general is a risk factor for cervical cancer, as an increase in cervical cancer is seen in HIV-positive women and women on cancer chemotherapy. More cases of cervical cancer are also noted in women with organ transplants who must take drugs that suppress their immune systems so that their bodies do not reject their transplanted organs.

In women who are not immunosuppressed, subtle immune system differences between women appear to be quite important. This poorly understood process is often referred to as "host factors" with the understanding that this ability varies from one woman ("host") to another. As an example, two women may have very similar backgrounds and sexual histories and both may be infected with the same type of HPV. One woman's immune system will efficiently fight her infection while the other's does not, leaving the way clear for the development of cervical cancer in five to ten years in the absence of proper medical care. Medical researchers are currently intensely interested in defining these mysterious "host factors."

WHICH AGE AND POPULATION GROUPS ARE MOST AT RISK FOR CERVICAL CANCER?

The bulk of our discussion thus far has focused on sexually active young women and their risk of acquiring HPV. The role of men and HPV will be addressed later in this chapter. A question asked by many women is whether HPV has the potential to stick around for many years. Will a woman infected in her teens or twenties, decades later, still harbor the virus? As we explained earlier, depending on a woman's "host factors," the virus may do one of several things. It may disappear entirely or it may persist and not cause any problems, in which case a woman may function as a carrier of HPV, passing it on to her sexual partners. Lastly, HPV may produce a precancer that can be detected on a Pap smear. In rare instances, it may produce a cancer with the potential to spread and kill. If a woman has had routine pelvic examinations with Pap smears, persistent HPV infections resulting in the presence of a cervical lesion would most likely have been detected and hopefully successfully treated.

There are, however, many women in the United States who do not have access to routine health care including regular Pap smears. It is estimated that 20 to 25 percent of American women have never been screened or are not routinely screened for cervical cancer. In studies which have asked why this happens, a number of barriers to Pap smear screening have been identified. A study conducted by the New Mexico Department of Health in 1998 identified cultural issues, fear of pain, fear of cancer, and embarrassment with the procedure. Other barriers include problems with transportation to clinic appointments and confusion about payment eligibility requirements. These women are often, but not exclusively, of low income and often of minority background.

While we certainly see cervical cancer in younger premenopausal women, probably the largest group of women diagnosed with cervical cancer today is older women between forty and seventy years of age, with poor access to health care. In contrast to our highly sexually active young women at risk for cervical cancer in the future, these older women generally are not very sexually active, but because of poor screening they form a substantial risk group for imminent development of the disease.

According to a 1996 National Cancer Institute publication, the highest rate of cervical cancer is seen in recent immigrants to this country, particularly Vietnamese and Korean women. Of nonimmigrant women, black, Hispanic, and Native American women develop cervical cancer at twice the rate found in white and Asian-American women. These are typically women who have not had a Pap smear in many, many years, if ever. There is also speculation that there are immune differences in different ethnic groups that can predispose them to SILs and cancer.

In the United States cervical cancer is a rare malignancy diagnosed in roughly 12,800 women a year resulting in about 5,000 deaths annually. Its presence elsewhere in the world, however, is staggering. It is the first or second most common malignancy of women in developing countries. The incidence of cervical cancer in parts of Africa and Asia is approximately ten times that of white women in the United States, and in Latin America it is approximately six times as high. This again reflects the powerful effect of poverty and the lack of healthcare programs that include Pap smear screening when considering the development of this disease. Women who emigrate from countries with a high rate of cervical cancer may continue to be at high risk for the disease. These women may face substantial barriers to cervical cancer screening due to problems with language and a lack of information about the availability of free or reduced-cost routine health care (Appendix B provides information on national programs offering low-cost or free Pap tests).

YOUR RISK OF DEVELOPING CERVICAL CANCER

Is it possible to assess your own cervical cancer risk? This is a difficult question to answer. However, a clinical test now exists to determine if you have the HPV virus in your cervix. But if you recall our discussion on the prevalence of HPV, you will remember that although many women are infected with this virus, few go on to develop cancer precursors or cancer. So just knowing if you are infected does not guarantee that you will develop cancer, and the absence of the virus by an HPV test does not release you from the responsibility of periodically having a Pap smear. (There are good uses for an HPV test and we will discuss them in chapter 5: "The Problem Pap Smear" and in chapter 9: "New Pap Smear Technologies.")

In fact, the "gold standard" for determining your chances of developing cervical cancer remains the Pap smear. A well-taken Pap smear, correctly interpreted, offers you the best chance of determining your future cervical cancer risks.

MEN AND HPV

Discussions about women, HPV infections, and cervical cancer are notorious for largely ignoring the subject of men and HPV infection. Why aren't men plagued with worries about genital precancers and cancers?

A number of researchers, including those at St. Thomas' Hospital in London in 1971, have established that women acquire their HPV infections almost exclusively from males who in turn have acquired HPV from either female or male sexual partners. HPV infections are seen in lesbian couples largely to the extent of the presence of any previous male partners. Men harbor HPV in multiple areas of their genitals such as the scrotum (the skin covering the testicles) and the penis. The virus is readily shed into shared genital secretions, from lubricating fluid to semen. The researchers at St. Thomas' Hospital verified that HPV is a highly infectious virus with a transmission rate from males to females estimated to range from 65 percent to much higher.

Despite the fact that men are reservoirs of HPV that can infect women, males are not routinely screened for HPV infection. A study from the University of California at Irvine in 1986 examined male partners of women with SILs and found HPV-associated lesions in almost 70 percent of the men. Detection of these lesions involves painting of a male's genitals with an acetic acid solution (essentially vinegar) which serves to highlight any HPV lesions. The male's genitals are then closely examined using a binocular-type instrument called a "colposcope," also used in examining a woman's cervix for HPV lesions. Depending on the type of HPV lesion, it may be removed using surgery, lasers, or topical medications. It is important to realize that removal of an HPV lesion may not always eradicate the infection, so a man may still be infectious after treatment.

Why isn't HPV detection and treatment of male partners undertaken? As a public-health measure, male sexual partners of women found to have other sexually transmitted diseases, such as gonorrhea and syphilis, are notified and treated, as required by law. In this way the spread of those diseases may be arrested. Why isn't this done for HPV, an infectious disease with cancer-producing potential?

The few studies that have looked at male treatment have concluded that treatment of male partners usually doesn't affect the course of their female partner's HPV problems. The vast majority of both men and women weather their HPV infections with no consequences other than passing the virus to their sexual partners. Clearly there is no point reporting to public-health authorities an infection which so many people carry with no ill effects and for which there is no real cure in terms of completely eradicating HPV from their bodies. Undoubtedly, it may also have a lot to do with men's (and probably physicians') unwillingness or squeamishness to dip a penis into vinegar, stare at it with a pair of binoculars, and then zap it with a burning laser.

There are some clinicians, however, who feel that male partners of women with HSIL should be examined and treated. Dr. Joel Palefsky, an expert in HPV infections in males, in a September 13, 1999, interview in the *New Yorker* magazine, describes these actively infected men as "a public-health risk to other women. . . ." He also points out that men who are infected with high-risk HPV can also endanger themselves. In the same way that cervical cancer in women is the end result of a long-standing infection by a high-risk HPV type, penile cancer appears to be the consequence of a similar infection in a male who is susceptible to the virus. Penile cancer, however, is an extremely rare tumor, occurring in fewer than 800 men a year in the United States, far less often than cervical cancer. These rare cancers typically arise on the penis glans or foreskin with spread to the shaft in advanced cases. While risk factors for penile cancer include sexual activity and HPV infection, more cases are seen in uncircumcised men than in circumcised. It is thought that poor genital hygiene contributes to this risk. Unluckily for women, the tissues of the female genital tract are much more vulnerable to the cancer-causing consequences of an HPV infection. The reason for this is currently unknown.

BACK TO KAREN

Before we leave this chapter, let's get back to our fictitious patient Karen in the examining room. She is now wondering how she managed to acquire a potentially deadly sexually transmitted virus since she has been monogamous throughout her eight-year marriage. Is this evidence that her husband has been sexually active with other women? While this is unfortunately always a possibility, keep in mind that HPV can have a long latency period: Karen's current HPV-related changes seen on her Pap smear may be the result of a latent infection she has harbored for years, one that has recently resurfaced. Currently, there is simply no way to tell.

If, like Karen, you are surprised to hear that cervical cancer is caused by a sexually transmitted virus, you are not alone. In a study done by Dr. Diane McGrory of Dedham, Massachusetts, when asked about the link between HPV and cervical cancer in an in-office survey, 73 percent of women were unaware that there was any relation between the two. We administered a similar survey to women awaiting their Pap smears in several suburban doctors' offices. Although the majority (93 percent) knew that Pap smears checked for cervical cancer, 68 percent of women did not know that HPV was the cause of cervical cancer. This is in spite of numerous media articles and public-health initiatives concerning HPV. Given the potentially devastating toll that an HPV infection can take on a woman's life, why isn't information on this virus and its consequences, in particular its sexual transmission, more widely known or appreciated?

One answer may be that information about HPV has been largely overshadowed by public-health information on HIV, another deadly virus. Another reason may be that even if information on this virus were more widely known, there is little that can be done to stop the infection short of abstinence from all sexual activity, a goal that we think is neither reasonable nor desirable. Even "safe sex" using condoms or engaging only in foreplay is not believed to prevent HPV infection. We know the virus is abundant in bodily secretions and has been shown to exist on scrotal skin, where it can be readily transferred to the women's vulva or external genitals, even without intercourse. Lastly, conversations about sexual health and the risks that one incurs with sexual activity have traditionally been difficult ones for physicians and their patients. We hope this book will help you better understand your risks for HPV infection and that it will provide you with some concrete steps to lessen the chances that you will develop cervical cancer.

With this introduction, let us now discuss what a Pap smear is all about, how it is obtained, and how it does its job in preventing cervical cancer. The next chapter will cover basics of your reproductive anatomy and how it relates to your Pap smear. We will guide you through a pelvic examination and the performance of the Pap test. You will follow a Pap smear through the laboratory where it is evaluated and finally to where you receive your Pap smear results.

T W O

Pap Smears 101

It might begin with a phone call from your doctor's office or with a post-card. The not-so-good news is that you have an abnormal Pap smear. If it is any comfort, millions of American women are in your shoes. If you are like the typical woman, an avalanche of worry descends the moment you receive this news. Whether you find out by phone or mail, most women are immediately filled with questions about this "atypical" result. How do we know this? In our combined nearly twenty years of cytology training and clinical practice, we have spoken to many women with abnormal Pap smears. Sometimes, all it takes is a chance mention by one of us that we look at Pap smears for a living to cause a near stranger to discuss her Pap smear concerns with us. More often, we are asked about a Pap smear diagnosis by a friend, colleague, or relative (or a friend of a colleague or a relative of a friend!). Underlying all these discussions are many unspoken questions: "What does this diagnosis really mean?" "What do I need to do next?" and "Am I at risk for developing cancer?"

We will be discussing the implications of your abnormal Pap smear in the chapters to follow, but first, it is important to have a good understanding of what your Pap test is all about. There has never been as much information about reproductive health available to the public as there is now. Ironically, we have still found that most women we speak with regarding their Pap smears are unsure about what their gynecologists are looking for in a pelvic exam or precisely why a Pap smear is performed. This is actually not very surprising because, unlike a male's reproductive organs which are constantly on display (at least for the owner's viewing pleasure), a woman's sexual organs are hidden from her. And except for a few embarrassing weeks in a coed sixth-grade health class or when something goes wrong, how many of us even think about our reproductive organs or remember what their varying functions are?

One of the goals of this chapter is to explain, in laywoman's language, what is happening while you are lying on your back straddled in stirrups in your gynecologist's office staring at the cracks in the ceiling. We will review the basic anatomy of a woman's sexual organs, and we will discuss the mysteries of the pelvic exam as well as the origins of the Pap smear, how it is performed, and what happens to your test. We will discuss the crucial subject of how errors occur in reading your Pap smear, and what the federal government mandates so that all such errors are kept to a minimum. We will also be discussing the limitations of the Pap test. Before you can understand what makes your Pap smear abnormal, it is important to understand how your test is performed and how it is interpreted.

THE FEMALE REPRODUCTIVE ORGANS

Most women are aware that the Pap smear is a test examining the cells of their cervix, but do you recall what and where your cervix is? Your cervix, along with your uterus, vagina, fallopian tubes, and ovaries are all organs having to do with reproduction and are collectively referred to as the female reproductive organs or female genitalia (figure 2-1). These are the organs which distinguish us from our male counterparts and enable us to become pregnant and bear children.

The "internal" female genitalia include the organs located inside your body—your vagina, cervix, uterus, fallopian tubes, and ovaries (figure 2-2). The vagina is the small chamber whose outer opening or "vulva," also known as the "labia" (the "external" genitalia), leads to the outside of a woman's body. You can feel the cervix at the back of your vagina as a firm, muscular doughnutlike structure. The dimple or depression in the middle of the cervix is the beginning of a connection or tunnel between the vagina and the inside of your uterus (figure 2-3). This narrow tunnel in the middle of the cervix is called the "endocervical canal." It is through this passage that menstrual

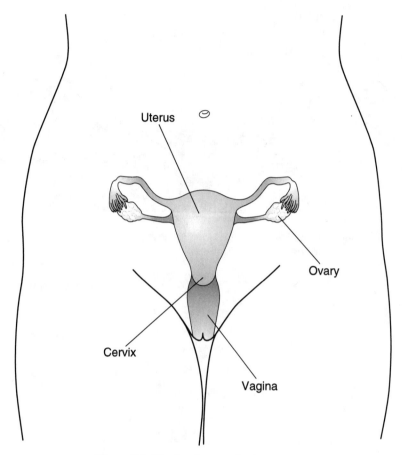

Figure 2-1. The female reproductive organs.

blood from the uterus flows outward and that male sperm travels upward to fertilize a female egg during conception. It is this tiny opening that widens amazingly during the birth process allowing delivery of a child.

During our reproductive lives, we are most aware of the uterus when its lining, also known as the "endometrium," breaks down and sheds every month as menstrual bleeding during our monthly periods. Its contractions can also be felt, mildly as menstrual cramping, and more intensely as contractions during labor. At the upper end of the uterus are two thin armlike projections, or fallopian tubes, extending to the left and right. On both sides, the fallopian tubes reach out toward a woman's two ovaries located to the left and right of the uterus. The ovaries are small organs, typically about the size

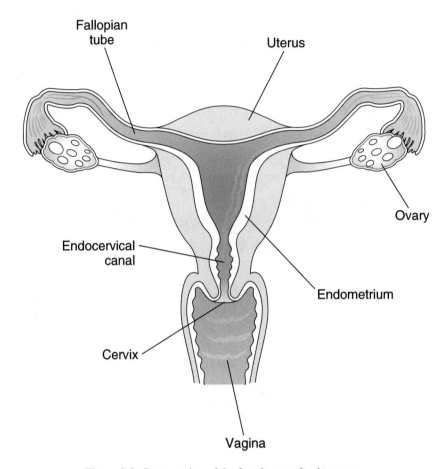

Figure 2-2. Cross section of the female reproductive organs.

of almonds, and are the site of egg production. The ovaries also produce most of the female hormones, namely, estrogen and progesterone.

The female reproductive organs are beautifully designed for their purpose of nurturing and bearing children. They are, however, all potential sites of cancer. One purpose of an annual pelvic examination is for your doctor or health practitioner to check these organs by feeling your uterus and ovaries to see if they have enlarged (one sign of a tumor) or feel tethered or "fixed" to the pelvis (another malignant feature). A healthy uterus with its attached fallopian tubes and ovaries should feel like they are "floating" to a clinician's examining hands. The examiner can also visualize the cervix, vagina, and

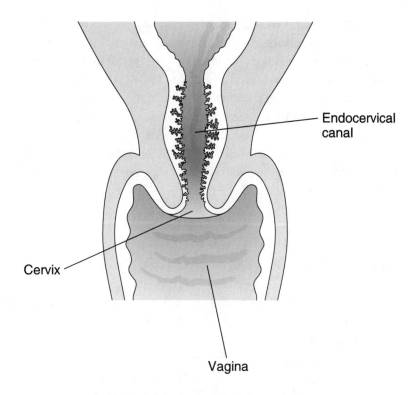

Figure 2-3. Cross section of the cervix.

vulva for abnormalities such as growths, areas of redness or roughness, or any lack of symmetry. The cervix and vagina are further investigated during the pelvic examination by the Pap test.

THE PELVIC EXAMINATION—HOW IS IT PERFORMED?

During a pelvic examination, a woman is situated on a nearly horizontal padded table which is equipped with "stirrups" for her feet. The stirrups look very similar to those on a saddle and the placement of a woman's feet in them allows for optimal positioning for the examination. This position, called the "lithotomy position," is very convenient for the person performing the examination but can leave a woman feeling rather vulnerable and uncomfortable. Because of this, some physicians will have a woman lie on her back without stirrups although the vast majority of doctors and clinics do use them. The clinician then will gently examine a woman's external genital tissues (her vulva) and then proceed with the insertion of a speculum. A speculum is an expandable metal or plastic device designed to be opened inside a woman's vagina. The speculum pushes apart the walls of the vagina so that it and the cervix can be seen. A Pap smear is then obtained from the cervix (details below). The pelvic examination then concludes with a "bimanual examination" whereby the clinician uses both hands, one gloved hand inside your vagina and the other pressing down on your abdomen, to feel your uterus and ovaries. By this technique, she is checking for any enlargement or unusual features of the pelvic organs that may signify a malignancy or other problems.

FOCUS ON THE CERVIX

Why is extra attention given to the cervix during a pelvic examination? As we saw in the previous chapter, the cervix is an organ that is highly susceptible to cancer. Of all the female reproductive organs, the cervix and nearby vagina are the most accessible for early cancer detection. While advanced cervical cancers may produce visible abnormalities on the cervix, or even symptoms such as bleeding, very early precancerous changes are happening at a microscopic level and are not visible to the naked eye. To detect these early changes, a test using a microscope is needed. This test is your Pap smear. Fortunately, using the test, cervical cancer is generally preceded by well-recognized cellular or microscopic changes which, if caught early, can be treated. Cervical cancer detection is truly one of "early detection." As we mentioned in the previous chapter, precancerous changes are also known as "precursor lesions," "cervical dysplasia," or "squamous intraepithelial lesions" (SILs). Along with full-blown cervical cancer, it is these precancerous changes that the Pap smear was designed to detect.

WHO INVENTED THE PAP TEST?

The Pap test was introduced in the 1940s by Cornell University scientist Dr. George Papanicolaou (1883–1962) as a method for detecting cervical cancer before women came to their doctors with advanced cancers. At that time, cervical cancer was a relatively common and greatly feared disease, being the number-one cancer killer of women. In the 1940s, 27 of every 100,000 women died of cervical cancer each year. Most of these women had cancers that were far advanced and incurable by surgery or other therapies when detected. The genius of Dr. Papanicolaou's test lay in its ability to detect changes in the cervix that occur before their transformation to cancer. These are changes that fall short of actual malignancy but indicate that a woman's cervix is on its way to becoming cancerous. Detecting these early precancerous changes allows a woman to be treated and cured before she develops a full-blown cancer.

Admittedly, the Pap test is not most women's idea of a fun way to spend an afternoon. From a public-health perspective, however, it is relatively easy to perform and is inexpensive to administer. These two features have made the Pap test very accessible to a large number of women. In fact, the Pap test has been widely utilized in most Western countries and is probably the most successful public-health test in medical history. Currently, only 8 women per 100,000 will die of cervical cancer, a dramatic drop in cervical cancer deaths since the inception of the Pap test. In the United States, cervical cancer is now the sixth most common cause of cancer deaths in women, ranking behind cancers of the lung, breast, colon, ovary, and pancreas.

HOW DOES THE PAP TEST WORK?

As we have mentioned, the Pap test functions by examining the cells of the cervix for changes that cannot be seen except under great magnification. Microscopically, the surface of the vagina and cervix are lined by a special type of tissue called the "squamous epithelium." This appears as alternating layers of flat tile-like squamous cells that fit together like bricks in a wall (figure 2-4). The cells all have a central dark dot or nucleus, which is where the cells' genetic material, or DNA, resides. The endocervical canal leading up into the uterus is lined by a different type of surface tissue called the "endocervical" or "glandular epithelium," which is thrown into gentle folds. These oblong cells appear like a picket fence with their nuclei pointing toward the bottom and their ample mucus-filled central portion (cytoplasm) pointing toward the top of the fence. As we will see later, subtle changes in the nucleus of either the squamous cells or endocervical cells can reflect pre-

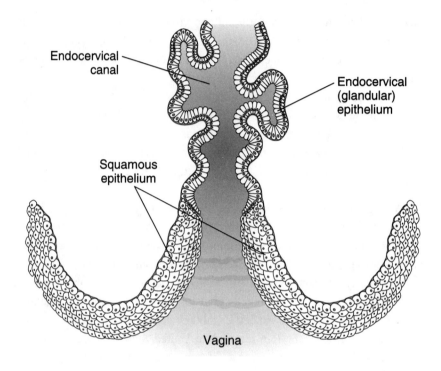

Figure 2-4. The tissues of the cervix.

cancerous changes. The area of the cervix where the squamous epithelium changes to glandular epithelium is known as the cervical "transformation" or "transition" zone (figure 2-5). Throughout its length the squamous and glandular epithelium is underlined by a structure called the "basement membrane." The purpose of the Pap test is to take samples of squamous and glandular cells at the transformation zone and examine them under a microscope for abnormalities indicating precancerous or cancerous changes.

The actual sampling of the cervix is performed by a gentle scraping of the surface of the cervix by special collection devices known as spatulas, brushes, and brooms. These devices come in various shapes and materials, typically either plastic or wood (figure 2-6). All of these devices are designed to collect the two types of cells present in the cervix (figure 2-7): (1) squamous cells from the squamous epithelium covering the smooth, rounded outer surface of the cervix and (2) glandular cells from the glandular epithe-

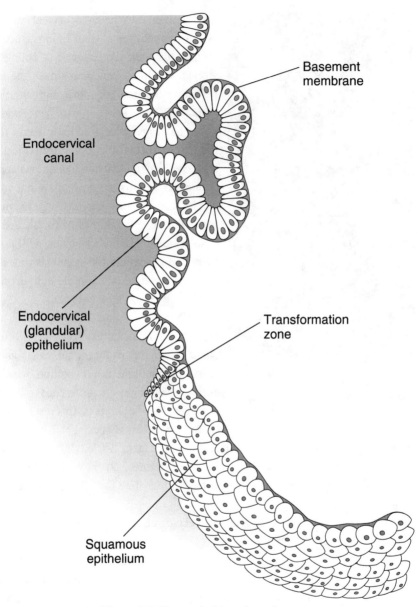

Figure 2-5. The cervical transformation zone.

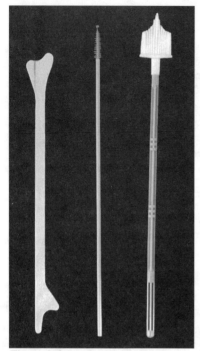

Figure 2-6. Instruments used for collecting a Pap smear (left to right): spatula, brush, broom.

lium high up into the endocervical canal. When scraped free of their linings, squamous cells look like large, flat cobblestones, while endocervical cells resemble kernels of corn with their nuclei pushed down toward one end. Since most precancers actually begin in the "transformation" or "transition" zone, it is crucial that both squamous and endocervical cells are present so that we can be sure that this area has been examined. Taking cell samples from this area is so critical that your Pap smear will not be read as adequate for diagnosis unless there is evidence that sample cells from this "zone" have been collected.

When performing a Pap smear on a woman, the clinician inserts one end of a spatula into the endocervical canal and twirls it around one full revolution, which allows the entire circumference of the outer cervix to be scraped. This results in a good sampling of squamous cells (figure 2-8). Next a special thin brush or broom is placed into the endocervical canal and again twirled 360 degrees to brush off the glandular cells that reside there (figure 2-9). Your clinician then spreads the cells they have collected onto a glass slide for subsequent microscopic examination.

A glass slide is a flat, rectangular piece of glass about the size of a stick of gum. Very simply, the material collected on the spatula and the brush are spread on one surface of a glass slide and the slide is very quickly "fixed" or preserved with an alcohol spray (figure 2-10). The alcohol fixation step is absolutely critical for a well-prepared Pap smear. It acts to instantly preserve the cells on the slide so that all the features of the freshly collected cells can be clearly seen using a microscope.

Prior to the actual collection of the cells, the glass slide is labeled on one end with the woman's name. This is the first in a long line of steps to assure proper identification of a woman's Pap smear and avoid possible mix-ups of

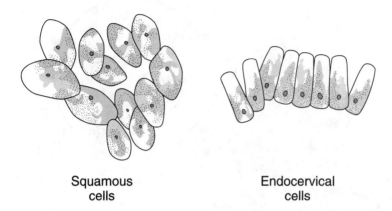

Squamous
cells

Endocervical
cells

Figure 2-7. Squamous and endocervical cells of the cervix as seen on a Pap smear.

slides between women. After the cells are collected, smeared on the labeled slide, and sprayed with fixative, the Pap smear is then placed in a protective cardboard or plastic holder for safe transport to the laboratory where the Pap smear will be evaluated. It is accompanied by paperwork with all pertinent patient information.

Your clinician who performed your pelvic examination and collected cells for your Pap smear will not be the one who examines it for precancerous or cancerous changes. Her job with the Pap smear is done until she has an actual Pap smear result or diagnosis to relay to you. The actual task of evaluating the cells on the slide is performed at a medical laboratory. The medical laboratory employs the behind-the-scenes healthcare workers who perform a wide variety of medical tests. For example, any of the many tests that can be performed on your blood are performed at a medical laboratory. Biopsies of various tissues from your body are prepared and diagnosed at a medical laboratory. Pap smears are also processed and interpreted here.

THE CYTOLOGY LABORATORY

The cytology laboratory is a specialized part of the medical laboratory, usually segregated in a quiet part of the lab so that the people who examine your cells can concentrate on this demanding task. "Cyto" is derived from the

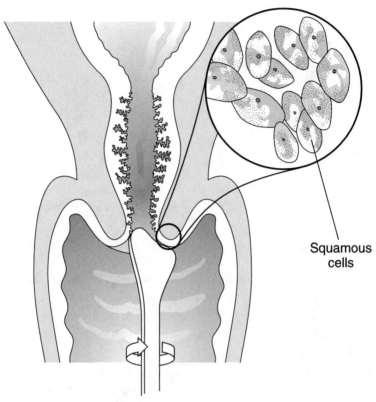

Squamous cells

Figure 2-8. Pap smear sampling of cervical squamous cells using a spatula.
Inset: Squamous cells as seen on a Pap smear.

Latin word meaning "cell" and this is one of the last remaining portions of
the lab where medical testing and interpretation is done by humans and not
by large automated machines. By far, the most common specimen examined
in the cytology laboratory is the Pap smear, but many other body sites lend
themselves to "cellular examination." Other cytology specimens include
urine, sputum, cerebral spinal fluids, and breast fluids, just to name a few. On
your slide's arrival at the cytology laboratory, the slide with its attendant
information will be entered or "accessioned" into the laboratory's information system and given a unique "accession number." The computer will also
check to see if you have had any previous Pap smears evaluated by the laboratory and if so, what those results were. All of this important information
will accompany your Pap smear during its evaluation.

As soon as your Pap smear has received an accession number, that

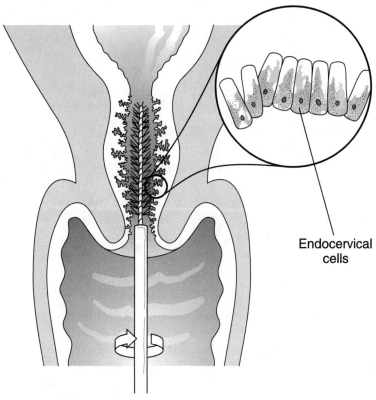

Endocervical
cells

Figure 2-9. Pap smear sampling of endocervical cells using a brush.
Inset: Endocervical cells as seen on a Pap smear.

number is recorded on the slide. At the moment, your specimen consists of a clear glass slide measuring about 3 inches by 1 inch with some cloudy white material spread on one surface. If someone were to look at your slide at this point through a microscope, they would see little more than a white haze. For your cells to be accurately assessed through a microscope, they need to be stained by special dyes. This is the next step in the processing of your Pap smear, staining by a special stain known as the Papanicolaou or Pap stain. This stain uses brilliant oranges, reds, and blues to color your squamous and glandular cells in a way that can be interpreted by cytologists. With the Pap stain, that central dot in the cell, or nucleus, becomes a pale cobalt to deep navy blue and details such as its shape, size, and depth of color can be studied. The material around the nucleus (the cytoplasm) becomes beauti-

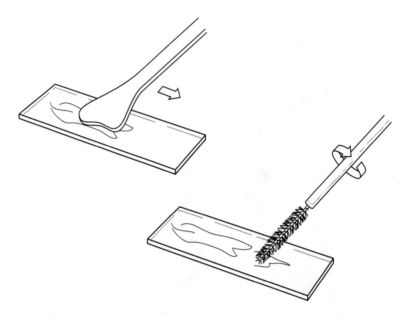

Figure 2-10. Preparation of a Pap smear with cervical cells spread on a glass slide.

fully translucent in candy shades of orange, pink, or blue. With its random array of jewel-like squamous and endocervical cells, a well-preserved and stained Pap smear can resemble a colorful work of abstract art.

CYTOTECHNOLOGISTS—
THE PRIMARY DIAGNOSTICIANS

The stained slides are then handed off to cytotechnologists who are the individuals involved in the "primary screening" of your Pap smear. Cytotechnologists are highly trained medical technologists who specialize in examining cells. As we mentioned, the vast majority of cytology involves analysis of Pap smears.

Cytotechnologists, however, are also trained to evaluate a wide variety of other cell specimens. The typical training of these specialists involves a Bachelor of Science degree that incorporates additional training in cytology from an accredited cytotechnology school. Each cytotechnologist is certified by the medical laboratory's certifying agency, the American Society of Clinical Pathologists. In our experience, cytotechnologists, with few exceptions, are highly motivated and dedicated individuals who take a great deal of professional pride in their occupation. They attend professional cytology meetings, have their own national organization (the American Society for Cytotechnology), and are instrumental in advancing the science of cytology through their participation in medical research and in the excellence of their day-to-day work.

Pap smear screening is the process whereby a cytotechnologist examines the entire surface of the Pap smear through a microscope. The microscope is equipped with special devices to hold a slide in place while every square millimeter of glass is examined by going back and forth across the slide. While it is obviously impossible to look at every cell on a slide, the vast majority of cells will be viewed and assessed by the cytotechnologist. This is an amazing feat considering the average Pap smear contains between 100,000 and 300,000 cells!

On viewing the cells on your slide, a cytotechnologist will decide several things. First of all, he or she will assess the slide for how well the cells were collected from your cervix and how useful the slide is for delivering a diagnosis. Are there enough squamous cells on the slide so that this Pap smear represents a well-sampled cervix? Are there enough endocervical cells present to indicate that cells from the transformation or transition zone were collected? Was the Pap smear fixed with alcohol promptly or is it air-dried and hence difficult to interpret? Is the slide free of excessive blood from a menstrual period or from a too vigorous scraping thus covering the cells to be viewed? Is inflammation from an infection obscuring the critical cells on the slide? The cytotechnologist runs through these questions with each slide screened. Depending on the answers to the above questions, the examiner may decide that your Pap smear is of marginal value for detecting cervical cancer or SILs. If this is the case, the cytotechnologist will indicate this on the report. With a suboptimal smear, your clinician may decide to repeat your Pap test.

The next task at hand is for the cytotechnologist to look for abnormal cells, either squamous cells from the outer cervix or glandular cells from the endocervical canal. As she views each cell on your slide, she will ask herself, "Is this cell normal or do I see any worrisome or abnormal changes?" If abnormalities are identified, the cells will be marked with marking pens. The cytotechnologist is also on the lookout for other changes: Is there evidence of an infection such as a yeast infection? Are the changes of pale glassy nuclei indicating a herpes infection present? Cervical squamous cells also reflect a woman's estrogen hormone status since estrogen causes predictable changes in these cells. A cytotechnologist can thus assess whether a woman is likely to still be having menstrual periods or if she is likely to be menopausal.

At the conclusion of this examination, the cytotechnologist will render a diagnosis. The vast majority of Pap slides will be acceptable in terms of having enough cells to view and in the visibility of those cells. Typically, over 90 percent of the slides will also be diagnosed as normal or "negative." This means that no abnormal changes are seen in either the squamous or glandular cells.

All of the cytotechnologist's observations will result in the formal Pap smear report. She will indicate that your specimen is "satisfactory for evaluation" and give a diagnosis with a statement like "Within normal limits" or "Negative for malignancy" indicating that no abnormalities are present. This means that your cervix has a very high likelihood of being free of disease and that you can wait another year for a repeat examination. With a normal Pap smear report, the likelihood of your having cervical cancer is very low although, as we will discuss below, a single Pap test cannot guarantee that you have no chance of having cervical cancer or of later developing cancer.

The next step is for the laboratory to generate a final report on paper with your Pap smear results. This report will be mailed or faxed to your doctor's or clinician's office whose personnel will then contact you with the results either by mail or by phone, although some offices do not contact patients with normal reports. The final report will be deposited in your medical record and also remain on record in the laboratory's report files.

A Pap smear with abnormal cells, however, is handled in a different manner. As mentioned above, abnormal cells are flagged by dots made with a marker pen on the slide for easy future reference. (Remember, there are about 200,000 cells on your Pap smear so it would be impossible to find a funny-looking cell twice without marking it!). All slides with abnormal cells are then routed to the pathologist for review.

PATHOLOGISTS: PHYSICIANS WHO DIAGNOSE ABNORMAL PAP SMEARS

A pathologist is a medical doctor who acts primarily as a consultant to other physicians and clinical staff in the interpretation of medical tests. He or she also runs the medical laboratory. They have completed hospital residency

Figure 2-11. Sources of error in evaluating Pap smears.

I. Pre-Laboratory Errors (While Pap Smear Obtained at Clinic)

Poorly Prepared Pap Smears
    Patient name not written on slide
    Poor fixation in alcohol
    Cells smeared too thickly
    Transformation zone not sampled
    Smear taken during menses with obscuring blood
    Smear taken during infection with obscuring inflammation

Inadequate Information on the Requisition Form
    Incorrect or missing patient name
    Incorrect or missing patient medical history
    Incorrect or missing patient birth date

II. Laboratory Errors (While Pap Smear at Cytology Laboratory)

Incorrect entry of patient information into laboratory computer system
    Patient name, birth date, last menstrual period, ordering physician,
    Numerical identifiers

Screening errors by cytotechnologists
    Abnormal cells not identified when present

Interpretative errors by cytotechnologists or pathologists
    Abnormal cells are identified but incorrectly interpreted

III. Post-Laboratory Errors (After Pap Smear Report Leaves Laboratory)

Pap smear completed and reported at laboratory but no report generated
    Computer system problem
Report mailed to physician but never received (lost in mail)
Report faxed to physician but never received
Result delivered to physician but not relayed to physician
    Report lost in physician's office or clinic
    Physician not informed by office personnel
Results mailed to patient from physician's office but never received by patient

programs in pathology, a process that typically takes five years after completion of medical school. Many of them have additional training known as
fellowships beyond their residencies. In many cytology laboratories, the
pathologists examining Pap smears will have done their fellowship training
in cytopathology so that they are, in essence, Pap smear "specialists." The
pathologist makes the final decision about any abnormalities detected by a
cytotechnologist's screening. Many of these slides with "abnormal" cells
will, on review by a pathologist, be felt to be truly benign in nature and the
slides reclassified as normal or benign. Other slides will be diagnosed as
having precancerous or cancerous changes. A minority of cases will be interpreted as "atypical," a diagnosis in between normal and a precancer. The
process of diagnosing abnormalities and the language of describing those
diagnoses will be discussed in further depth in chapter 3.

SOURCES OF ERROR IN THE CYTOLOGY LABORATORY

As you can see, your Pap smear takes a long trip starting with the collection
of cervical cell samples in your doctor's office to being accessioned and
stained in the cytology laboratory, through its final screening process by the
cytotechnologists with possibly a further look by a pathologist. The result, of
course, is a Pap smear report with you being notified of the results. At any
one of these steps, there are opportunities for errors, which are not good in a
cytology laboratory because the consequences can be so dire. Much of the
daily work in the cytology laboratory and in your clinician's office revolves
around keeping the number of errors to a minimum. Unfortunately, they still
occur and you should be aware of their sources.

It is helpful if we sort errors into three general types (figure 2-11):

1. *Pre-laboratory errors* occur at your doctor's office at the time she
   conducts your Pap test. These errors relate to Pap smear collection,
   preparation, slide labeling, delivery to the lab, and preparation of a
   Pap smear requisition form.

2. *Laboratory errors* are those relating to entry into the laboratory computer system, slide staining, laboratory labeling, cytotechnologist
   screening, and pathologist interpretation.

3. *Post-laboratory errors* are those relating to generating the final report with final delivery of that report to you.

If we look first at pre-laboratory errors occurring at your doctor's office, the most common ones seen are poorly prepared Pap smears which are not promptly fixed in alcohol. Since a variety of medical specialists may perform Pap smears, they may not all have received optimal training and instruction in the proper way to perform a Pap smear, including its fixation. The resulting air-dried Pap smears will contain cells with nuclei that are enlarged and irregular. As we will see in the next chapter, these are both features of abnormal cells but in this case they are purely a result of poor fixation. We will discuss other causes of "limited" and "unsatisfactory" Pap smears in subsequent chapters. Clinicians who have chronic "air-drying" problems may benefit from obtaining Pap smears through the use of the newer liquid-based Pap tests (see chapter 9 for a discussion of these tests).

Another common pre-laboratory error is an incomplete Pap smear requisition form, one that omits important patient history such as previous abnormal Pap smears, previous treatment for abnormal Pap smears, and date of the last menstrual period. It is also important to let the laboratory know if a patient is "high-risk" since most labs have special quality control mechanisms for cases from women in this category. This high-risk group would include women with previous abnormal Pap smears, multiple sexual partners, and those who have contracted sexually transmitted diseases such as gonorrhea, chlamydia, or syphilis.

Seen uncommonly as a pre-laboratory error are mislabeled Pap smear slides, that is, a slide labeled with one woman's name but attached to a Pap smear requisition with another woman's name. This latter error will quickly prompt a call to the doctor's office and may well result in both women coming back into the office for a repeat Pap smear. Pap smears that leave the doctor's office without a patient name written on one end are considered unacceptable by the laboratory and usually result in the test needing to be repeated. Delivery of Pap smear slides to a cytology laboratory is usually problem-free; however, slides can be lost or broken. Failure of a clinician to properly use a protective holder can result in Pap smear slide breakage and again, the need to repeat the test.

Laboratory errors involve the many steps and stops your Pap smear takes once received by the cytology laboratory. First, let's look at "accessioning" errors where the information listed on each patient's Pap smear requisition form is entered into the laboratory's computer. Whether it's the wrong patient name, date of birth, past medical history, date of last menstrual period, the ordering physician, billing information—you name it—there is always the chance that it can be entered into the computer incorrectly. Most of these errors are easily caught and corrected, however, the most serious errors are ones involving patient names. From the first to the last, laboratory personnel handling your Pap smear have the responsibility to check and recheck names on paperwork against names on Pap smears to catch any errors as early as possible. Most labs have elaborate systems for catching identification errors.

Errors occurring during the process of Pap smear screening by cytotechnologists have certainly garnered more than their fair share of media attention. First, let's gain an understanding of the Herculean task of screening a Pap smear. As mentioned previously, each Pap smear slide has on average 200,000 individual cells smeared across its surface. The cytotechnologist's job is to screen sixty to eighty or so of these slides each day and decide whether they look normal or not. It is an accepted fact that some abnormal cells will be missed by a cytotechnologist's eyes. Although this would seem to be a disaster, in the vast majority of cases, the significance of these "missed cells" is not immediately life threatening for the following reason. Cervical cancer progression is generally a slow process taking years from the first diagnosis of precancer to that of full-blown cervical cancer. Consequently, even if an early precursor is missed on Pap smear screening, in theory a patient will have several years' worth of Pap smears to catch the SIL before it progresses to cancer. For this reason, it is vital to have regular Pap smear screenings since the full power of this exam is only realized when you have had a normal result for several years in a row.

We are in no way downplaying the realities of these "missed" Pap smears. In the last decade or so, there have been several advances in Pap smear screening technologies that have helped to address the issues of missed abnormal cells. Furthermore, we now know that in some women cervical cancer progresses more rapidly so that there is less time in which to discover a cancer. Some women, particularly those who fall into high-risk categories for the development of cervical cancer, may be interested in these newer technologies. We will address these advances and their benefits and drawbacks in chapter 9.

The last area of laboratory error centers around the pathologist's interpretation of any abnormal cells identified by the cytotechnologist. As we will see in chapter 3, the interpretation of atypical cells can be exceedingly difficult and can be very subjective. In addition, pathologists are sometimes called upon to make a diagnosis on as few as one or two cells out of the hundreds of thousands of cells on a slide. This difficult task can lead to interpretive errors, which is why all atypical reports, even those suggestive of a benign process, must be followed up by a repeat normal Pap smear before a woman can be given a clean bill of health.

Post-laboratory errors revolve around making sure each woman gets her Pap smear result. These errors will result from any problems with a laboratory's report-printing operation, mail delivery service, fax machines, or office personnel who don't relay results to doctors or to patients. Most cytology laboratories will, on a monthly basis, send to each doctor's office or clinic a list of all of their patients who have received an atypical Pap smear report. The doctor's office can then verify receipt of those Pap smear reports. Some cytology laboratories will also call a clinic or office with the results from any Pap smear showing cervical cancer or a serious precancerous lesion.

HOW THE GOVERNMENT
REDUCES ERRORS WITH PAP SMEARS

On November 2, 1987, an article in the *Wall Street Journal* investigated abuses of so-called Pap smear mills—laboratories where many more Pap smears were being read on a daily basis than is now considered safe. These readings were also done under questionable conditions with some labs engaging in sloppy practices. Because of this increased attention to Pap smears and the heightened appreciation of the potential for errors, the federal government enacted legislation to reduce Pap smear errors to a minimum. This legislation, which was passed in the early 1990s, is entitled the Clinical Laboratory Improvement Act of 1988, otherwise known as CLIA '88. While directed at pathology laboratories as a whole, many of the provisions of this legislation are quite specific for Pap smears. They chiefly address the laboratory errors discussed above, such as screening or interpretation errors of abnormalities seen on Pap smear slides. The following describes some of the CLIA '88 provisions which are in place in every cytology laboratory in this country:

1. **10 percent slide rescreen:** Each day, every cytotechnologist will have 10 percent of the slides she called normal rescreened by another cytotechnologist or pathologist. In most laboratories, the 10 percent figure is a minimum figure with many laboratories rescreening 20 percent or higher of normal Pap smears. In general, Pap smears from all high-risk women are also rescreened. This rescreening is done prior to issuing a final report on a Pap smear. The point of rescreening Pap smears is to catch early, prior to patient notification, any Pap smears with abnormal cells which have been missed by the screening cytotechnologist. Such incorrectly diagnosed Pap smears are called "false negative Pap smears" (the Pap smear is "falsely" called negative or normal). This practice is also an excellent way to keep close tabs on all cytotechnologists. Any cytotechnologist who may be having problems screening with a high degree of accuracy can be quickly recognized. Problem cytotechnologists, although rare, do occur and since the laboratory has the first priority of high-quality patient care, this problem has to be dealt with quickly. Once recognized, cytotechnologists with screening problems may then have more of their daily Pap smears rescreened, may be asked to screen fewer slides each day, or may need more comprehensive in-service instruction and even cytology retraining.

2. **Five-year look-back:** This CLIA '88-mandated practice requires a review of all previously diagnosed negative Pap smears for any woman who has a newly diagnosed cervical cancer or HSIL. In this way, a laboratory can recognize screening or interpretation errors (again, false negative Pap smears), and perhaps even recognize problem cytotechnologists and pathologists.

3. **Pap smear and cervical biopsy correlation:** After a Pap smear has been called abnormal, a woman may end up having a cervical biopsy to confirm this diagnosis. This involves removing a tiny piece of cervical tissue to be examined under a microscope. This biopsy will also be given a diagnosis by a pathologist (see chapter 4 for a further discussion of cervical biopsies and other diagnostic tests of the cervix). This CLIA '88 provision requires that the laboratory compare a woman's original abnormal Pap smear with the cervical biopsy to make sure the diagnoses of these two samples agree. In this way, laboratories can catch Pap smears that are incorrectly diagnosed as a precancer or SIL when they are actually normal (false positive Pap smears).

THE PAP TEST IS NOT A PERFECT TEST

CLIA '88 also addresses other aspects of cytology laboratories to ensure that Pap smears are handled in as error-free a manner as possible. Even with these federal laws in place and even with the best of intentions, errors may happen in the very best of cytology laboratories. It is quite difficult for the public to embrace the concept of "acceptable error" or "minimum acceptable error" in medical testing. It is important to keep in mind, however, that unlike many other examples of medical testing that rely on large automated machines, a Pap smear is still a test involving interpretations by human eyes of sometimes very subtle cellular changes. As such, it is not surprising that this test is not 100 percent foolproof in detecting cancerous and precancerous changes. There have been recent developments in automating Pap smear screening but even the "machine-screened" slides ultimately need human eyes to judge abnormal cells. These are discussed in chapter 9.

Fortunately, part of the genius of the Pap test is how well it fits with the nature of cervical cancer. An essential part of the Pap test is that a woman must have one on a regular basis if the test is to be successful. Though Dr. Papanicolaou's test is an excellent one it is still not perfect. By its very nature, some abnormal cells on a Pap smear may be missed by the screening process. Remember, the cytotechnologist is reviewing hundreds of thousands of cells. Cervical cancer and precancers, however, tend to grow rather slowly so that if abnormal cells are missed one year, they will probably be seen the next year without any harm being done to the patient. Problems arise when women do not schedule their annual pelvic examinations. Most cases of cervical cancer today occur in women who have either never had a Pap test or have gone more than five years since their last examination. It is clear that efforts to further reduce the incidence of cervical cancer in women needs to focus on encouraging all women to have an annual Pap test as we continue to work on improving the test itself.

The previous two chapters have provided important information on why Pap smears are critical for the prevention of cervical cancer and details on how the test is performed. In the next chapter we will provide information allowing you to become better informed about your Pap smear. By learning how to read your Pap smear report, you will gain the tools necessary to understand your Pap smear results and to ask meaningful questions of your clinician.

T H R E E

How to Read Your Pap Smear Report

In the past, if you received an abnormal Pap smear report, there was really nothing you could do other than wait and worry until your next gynecologic exam, which might be months away. Our experience is that most women want and need information about their abnormal results during this anxious time. They have a strong desire to understand these abnormalities, their chances for subsequently developing cancer, and how the diagnosis impacts their future sexual and reproductive health.

We recognize that very few women actually see their Pap smear reports. If your clinician is able to communicate your results to you in a way that is understandable, reading your own report may not be necessary. Many women, however, want more information than their doctor's office can provide. For these women, we offer this chapter to assist you in understanding Pap smear diagnoses.

Although these reports, like any other medical document, are written by doctors and are chock-full of medical jargon, we will show you what to look for, when to worry, and when to ask for a repeat smear. We will explain the major diagnostic categories and the all-important concept of "adequacy." Lastly, we will explore the aggravating "atypical" category, which is neither normal nor clearly diagnostic for a cancer or precancer. With this information, every woman can more fully understand her Pap smear report and use that information to decide on her next course of action.

Figure 3-1. Sample Pap smear report.

Patient Name:	Wendy Woman	Date of Birth: 1/1/60
Requesting Physician:	Joan Smith, M.D.	
Date Ordered:	1/1/01	
Medical Record Number:	00001	

GYNECOLOGIC CYTOLOGY (PAP SMEAR REPORT)

HISTORY:

Clinical: Annual Examination

Last Menstrual Period: 12/15/00

GYN: History of ASCUS Pap smear

Indication: History of ASCUS 5/98 and 8/96

High Risk?: Yes

MATERIAL SUBMITTED: Cervical and vaginal smear

SPECIMEN ADEQUACY: Satisfactory for evaluation
An endocervical component is present

DIAGNOSIS: Atypical Cells of Undetermined Significance, Favor
Low-Grade Squamous Intraepithelial Lesion

Screened by:	Cynthia Cytotech, Cytotechnologist
Verified by:	Patricia Pathologist, M.D.
Date Reported:	1/05/01

THE PAP SMEAR REPORT FORMAT

Every Pap smear taken from a woman results in a Pap smear report. Each of these reports must contain by government mandate certain essential pieces of information. Although all reports contain basically the same information, Pap smear reports from different laboratories may look somewhat different. As we alluded to in the last chapter, your Pap smear report can be broken down into two important sections mirroring the two tasks of the cytotechnologist as

---

Figure 3-2. Terms of Pap smear adequacy.

Satisfactory for Evaluation

Satisfactory for Evaluation but Limited by:
> Marginal number of squamous cells
> Inadequate number of endocervical cells
> Poorly fixed or preserved cells
> Obscuring blood, inflammation, or mucus
> Thickly smeared cells

Unsatisfactory for Evaluation
> Insufficient number of squamous cells
> Cells virtually obscured by blood, inflammation, thickly smeared cells

---

she screens your slide. These two sections are: (1) Statement of Pap smear adequacy and (2) Diagnosis. Figure 3-1 contains a sample Pap smear report.

PAP SMEAR ADEQUACY

Your Pap smear report will contain a statement commenting on the quality of the specimen, also called its "adequacy." This is a crucial statement that lets you and your physician know if your Pap smear is of high enough quality to even render a reliable diagnosis. There are a number of features that comprise a quality or "adequate" Pap smear. If a Pap smear is of poor quality for any of the reasons discussed below, any diagnosis given is likely to be unreliable as well. Clinicians may recommend that a suboptimal Pap smear be repeated.

There are three categories of adequacy used in Pap smear reporting. These are: (1) satisfactory for evaluation (adequate), (2) unsatisfactory for evaluation (inadequate), and (3) satisfactory but limited for evaluation (marginally adequate). One of these three categories will be found on your Pap smear report, typically toward the top or the bottom of the report following a heading such as "Specimen Adequacy."

What determines if your Pap smear is satisfactory for evaluation? There are actually a number of criteria which must be met as we will discuss below and are summarized in figure 3–2.

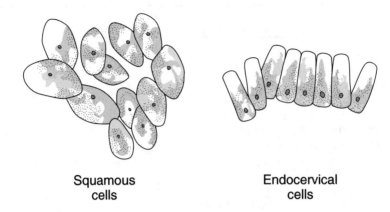

Squamous
cells

Endocervical
cells

Figure 3-3. Squamous and endocervical cells of the cervix as seen on a Pap smear.

NUMBER OF SQUAMOUS CELLS

First and foremost, were there enough cells taken from your cervix? In other words, did your clinician do an adequate job of sampling the cervix when obtaining your Pap smear? You may recall from chapter 2 that two types of cells should be present on your Pap smear: squamous cells and endocervical (glandular) cells (figure 3–3). The guideline used by American laboratories is that squamous cells (these are the large, flat cells that look like cobblestones or polygonal tiles) must cover at least 10 percent of the slide's surface in order to be considered satisfactory for evaluation.

PRESENCE OF ENDOCERVICAL CELLS

A Pap smear generally has many more squamous cells than endocervical or glandular cells. Far fewer endocervical cells (the cells which resemble kernels of corn, figure 3–3) are required to call a Pap smear "satisfactory." Recall, however, that endocervical cells are the "marker" or sign that cells have been taken from the all-important transformation or transition zone, the primary site of HPV infection in the cervix. Endocervical cells can also be replaced by "squamous metaplasia" which is a modified endocervical cell found at the transformation zone. At least a few groups of endocervical or squamous metaplastic cells should be present. The complete absence of them would cause us to call a Pap smear "satisfactory but limited" due to a lack of evidence that the transformation zone was sampled.

The absence of endocervical cells may reflect poor technique on the part of the person obtaining your Pap smear. In some groups of women, however, the absence of endocervical cells in a Pap smear is not unusual and is actually expected. A woman who has previously had her uterus surgically removed (hysterectomy) will generally not have any endocervical cells left to sample on a Pap smear because the cervix is often removed along with the uterus. With their cervixes removed, these women will have Pap smears taken from their vaginas, which are still susceptible to HPV infection and cancer. Older women well into their menopause often will not have endocervical cells on their Pap smears because of changes in their cervixes which occur with age. As a woman grows older, her transformation zone may ascend high into her endocervical canal so it is difficult to reach when collecting her Pap smear. Postmenopausal women will sometimes experience a tight narrowing of the endocervical canal so that the canal is not easily sampled during a routine Pap smear.

Pregnant women are another group of women who may have no endocervical cells on their Pap smears. Aggressive sampling high into the endocervical canal is not recommended during pregnancy due to concerns about disturbing a woman's pregnancy. After all, an important function of the cervix is for the endocervical canal to stay tightly shut during pregnancy so the fetus will stay in the uterus.

In any of the above situations, the lack of endocervical cells usually still allows a Pap smear to be considered "satisfactory." If the Pap smear is called "satisfactory but limited," for example, during pregnancy, your clinician (and you) will understand that this is an acceptable reading for you.

CELL VISIBILITY

Another important consideration in assessing your Pap smear for adequacy is how well the cells can be seen. Obviously, if the critical cells on a Pap smear are obscured by blood, mucus, and inflammation, all of which are commonly present in a woman's cervix, it will be very difficult to make a diagnosis. We can only diagnose what we can see! By inflammation we mean the white blood cells in your body that gather to fight infection. Very often, inflammatory cells will reside in the cervix without an identifiable cause or infection.

However, occasionally, an infectious agent such as yeast or the parasite Trichomonas will be seen and reported on your Pap smear. (Common infections of the cervix are discussed in chapter 8). If greater than 75 percent of the cells present are obscured by blood, inflammation, or mucus, your Pap smear is regarded as unsatisfactory with the reason stated on the report. If somewhere between 50 percent and 75 percent of the cells cannot be seen, the Pap smear is called "satisfactory but limited for evaluation" with the obscuring factors mentioned in the report.

"Air-drying artifact" is another very common reason for Pap smear inadequacy, as mentioned previously. Recall this is due to poor cell preservation and can be directly traced to the clinic personnel preparing the slide at the time of your Pap smear. This usually reflects less-than-optimal technique when acquiring a Pap smear, although in some instances air-drying can be related to patient factors (e.g., in postmenopausal women who may have a lack of sufficient lubrication). For optimal preservation, the cells taken from your cervix and placed on a glass slide need immediate preservation or fixation with alcohol or fixative spray. Immediate means just that; the slide should be sprayed within seconds of the cells being smeared on the slide. Any delay will result in cells drying up on the slide where they can then appear grotesquely enlarged with apparent irregularities. These features can appear quite alarming and can be confused with true abnormalities of the cervix. Among some doctors' practices, air-dried Pap smears are a common cause of atypical Pap smears.

What should be done after a "satisfactory," "satisfactory but limited," and "unsatisfactory" Pap smear? For an unequivocal "satisfactory" Pap smear, the diagnosis given should be considered reliable and further decisions about courses of action can be confidently made by you and your clinician.

For a "satisfactory but limited" Pap smear, there is an implication that the diagnosis may not be entirely reliable. If limited due to some obscuring factor such as inflammation or blood, this means that the diagnosis given applies to the cells that were visible but all bets are off about the cells that were not clearly seen. Many clinicians will be uncomfortable with this and will suggest that you come back in a few months to try and obtain a better, more visible Pap smear prior to one year. However, if you are a woman with a long history of normal Pap smears and you are in a long-term monogamous relationship, this may not be felt to be necessary. If your Pap smear was limited due to inflammation from a recognized infection, you should have your infection treated prior to a repeat Pap smear. A Pap smear that is limited due to the absence of endocervical cells implies that the transformation zone was not sampled. Clinicians will sometimes want to repeat those Pap smears, particularly if the woman has had a record of previous abnormal smears.

A Pap smear that is "unsatisfactory" is exactly that. No diagnosis will be given on an unsatisfactory Pap smear. The report will state "unsatisfactory for evaluation" along with the reason. This statement requires that a clinician call a woman back in for a repeat Pap smear within a few months and is essentially equivalent to no Pap smear having been taken at all. If your Pap smear is called "unsatisfactory," you should make an appointment to repeat the test.

DIAGNOSIS

This is the place on the report where the medical opinion on your Pap smear is recorded. This section is typically set off from the rest of the report, sometimes in bold type, by the heading "Diagnosis" or "Interpretation" or "Findings." The actual diagnosis will use specific medical phrases and terminology and will tell you if any abnormalities of the cervix were seen. This will dictate what your future medical treatment or follow-up should be.

Before we get into the diagnostic terminology, let's first remind ourselves that the foremost goal of a Pap smear is to detect changes in your cells that indicate current or past infection by the human papillomavirus or HPV. As we know, the medical term for an HPV-related precancerous cervical lesion is a squamous intraepithelial lesion or SIL, also known as "dysplasia." Sometimes we can be absolutely sure that we are seeing signs of a SIL. These cellular changes, however, are not always clear-cut and pathologists may see changes that aren't absolutely conclusive for a SIL but still make us worry that a SIL might be present. An important point, which we will come back to, is that *there are other, innocuous causes of abnormal cells on a Pap smear that do not indicate precancerous changes.* Therefore, an abnormal Pap smear is not always evidence for the presence of HPV effects and does not always mean that a patient is at increased risk for later developing cervical cancer.

THE BETHESDA SYSTEM

The terminology used in Pap smear evaluations has undergone several changes since Dr. Papanicolaou's original classification system. The current system most in use in the United States was established in 1988 and is known as the Bethesda System (figure 3-4). Some doctors and labs still refer to cervical lesions by their old terminology. To help you make sense of these various synonyms for cervical diagnoses, figure 3-5 compares the various systems for describing precancerous lesions of the cervix.

The Bethesda System of Pap smear terminology derived in 1988 is still in use in 2001. In May 2001, however, a conference was held to discuss changes to the 1988 Bethesda System. As of publication time, these changes have not yet been formally released but will be sometime in 2001. We most likely will see some new terms for Pap smear diagnoses in the near future. In particular, the category of Atypical Cells of Undetermined Significance (ACUS) and Benign Cellular Changes (BCC) may be modified.

"NORMAL" AND "BENIGN CELLULAR CHANGES"

What Pap smear diagnoses might you see on your Pap smear report? The first, of course, is everyone's favorite diagnosis (yours as well as ours): "within normal limits" or "negative." These diagnoses mean the same thing: your Pap smear shows no abnormalities. Usually this diagnosis means that you don't need to return to your physician or clinic for a year. Although your Pap smear may carry a "normal" diagnosis, recall that it still may be considered "satisfactory for evaluation but limited" for some reason, which will be stated on your report. As mentioned above, some clinicians feel uncomfortable if you have a "satisfactory but limited" statement in your report. Depending on your history, they may have you return for a repeat Pap smear earlier than one year. The vast majority of Pap smears (over 90 percent) are normal.

Another diagnosis you may run across is that of "benign cellular changes," also known as "BCC." This is a Pap smear that is normal but shows mild changes in the squamous or endocervical cells which fall short of being worrisome for a SIL. Usually this means that some nuclei are just a little darker or are slightly more irregular than we normally see. Such benign changes may reflect changes in your cervical cells from infections such as yeast or the parasite Trichomonas. These changes are also known as "reactive" or "reparative" changes. If a specific infection is identified on your Pap smear with a "BCC" diagnosis, your physician may want to put you on treatment to clear it up, such as an antifungal cream for a yeast infection. As with a "negative" diagnosis, a "BCC" diagnosis means you will not need to return for a repeat Pap smear until your next yearly checkup.

ATYPICAL SQUAMOUS CELLS OF
UNDETERMINED SIGNIFICANCE (ASCUS)

It is with this ambiguous diagnosis that the problems with Pap smears begin. An "atypical" report refers to a Pap smear that is not normal but also does not have features of a clear-cut SIL or precancer. It is a diagnosis that lives in a very murky zone between normal and a firm diagnosis of a precancerous lesion. Atypical Pap smears are given the official (and unhelpful) designation of "atypical squamous cells of undetermined significance" or "ASCUS" (pronounced "ask us"). Medical personnel will often refer to your atypical Pap smear as an "ASCUS." This is shorthand for "we just can't tell."

Recall that on a Pap smear slide viewed under a microscope, squamous cells look like polygonal tiles with central dark blue dots which are the nuclei containing your genetic material. The squamous cells seen in an atypical Pap smear may have nuclei that are somewhat larger than normal. The guideline of 2.5 times larger than a normal squamous cell nucleus is frequently used. The nuclei of atypical squamous cells may also be darker than normal or perhaps more irregular or wrinkly in their outline (think of raisins) (figure 3-6). The atypical cells are usually surrounded by numerous normal cells so that we can make these comparisons. The changes are also much greater in degree than we would expect in a reactive case which we would diagnose as a benign cellular change (BCC). All of these features: increase in the nuclear size, darkness, and irregularity are all changes which, if present to an extreme degree, are part of the diagnosis of a SIL. In an atypical Pap smear, some but not all of these features are present or the features are present in just a few cells. In short, the pathologist reading your slide feels that the evidence present is just too scanty to merit a SIL diagnosis.

The number of atypical cells on an atypical Pap smear will vary, but as few as a single atypical cell (particularly if it is markedly atypical) can be enough to push your Pap smear out of the "normal" category and into the anxiety-ridden world of the atypical Pap smear. The concern with atypical cells is that while they might not be diagnosable as a SIL on this particular Pap smear, they may reflect the early stages of a SIL, or perhaps one that is very small and was just barely sampled when your Pap smear was taken.

How valid is all this worry about a precancer in just a few slightly funny-looking atypical cells among the hundreds of thousands of normal cells? Since these cells don't readily resemble a SIL, how often do they truly predict a future or present precancerous lesion? A number of studies have followed women with ASCUS diagnoses to see how many later end up with SILs or cervical precancers. The numbers vary from study to study but somewhere between 30 to 40 percent of women with atypical Pap smears will later prove to have a SIL. A small proportion of these women will later be shown to have a high-grade SIL. Remember, HSILs are the lesions that have the greatest potential to progress to cancer.

Are there other causes, apart from HPV-related changes, that can lead to an atypical Pap smear? Absolutely. Infections such as yeast or the parasite Trichomonas, for example, can enlarge the cell's nucleus, or cause it to look dark or irregular. These infections usually display other changes on a Pap smear that accompany a reactive process, such as numerous inflammatory cells. But in other instances, these infections will be more subtle and not clearly recognized as infections.

The mere presence of reactive changes will not automatically make a Pap smear "atypical." Pathologists are familiar enough with reactive cell changes that we generally will describe a reactive Pap smear as having "benign cellular changes" (see above) simply because we have become familiar over time with the cell changes associated with a reactive process. It is when the changes surpass our "reactive" threshold that a test result is called "atypical." This diagnosis reflects our uncertainty in the cellular changes that we see. The cells look atypical although we cannot conclusively diagnose a precancerous process. If all of this sounds subjective, it's because it is. Diagnosing atypias on a Pap smear often involves more of the "art" than the "science" of medicine.

Women on contraceptive hormones, especially Depo-Provera or Norplant, may also have changes on their Pap smears which are difficult to call normal, even when we know women are taking these medications. Another problem area is with women who have just delivered a baby and who are per-

Figure 3-4. Pap smear diagnoses:
The Bethesda System for classifying cervical smears.

Within Normal Limits

Benign Cellular Changes
    Infection
          Trichomonas vaginalis
          Fungal infection such as *Candida* (yeast)
          Bacterial vaginosis
          Herpes simplex virus
          Actinomyces

    Reactive Changes
          Inflammation (includes repair changes)
          Atrophy with inflammation (atrophic vaginitis)
          Radiation effects
          Intrauterine contraceptive device (IUD)

Epithelial Cell Abnormalities
    Squamous Cells:
          Atypical Squamous Cells of Undetermined
          Significance (ASCUS)
          Low-Grade Squamous Intraepithelial Lesion (LSIL)
          High-Grade Squamous Intraepithelial Lesion (HSIL)
          Squamous Cell Carcinoma
    Endocervical Cells:
          Atypical Glandular Cells of Undetermined
          Significance (AGUS)
          Endocervical Adenocarcinoma
          Endometrial Adenocarcinoma

haps breastfeeding. After childbirth women typically visit their clinic for a checkup including a Pap smear six weeks after delivery. In a small fraction of these women, their Pap smears may show atypical changes due to being recently pregnant.

Older women who are in menopause may also have atypical Pap smears. In all of these examples, we are looking at women with a different hormone status than your typical woman of childbearing age receiving a Pap smear. In many instances, we suspect that the atypical changes are due to the hormonal changes but we cannot be absolutely sure. An "ASCUS" diagnosis will result. We will discuss some of these "special" atypical instances in chapter 5 on the

Figure 3-5. Comparison of diagnostic names for squamous cervical lesions.

Low-Grade Squamous Intraepithelial Lesion (LSIL)
> Mild or Slight Dysplasia
> Cervical Intraepithelial Neoplasia 1 (CIN 1)

High-Grade Squamous Intraepithelial Lesion (HSIL)
> Moderate or Severe Dysplasia
> Carcinoma In-Situ
> Cervical Intraepithelial Neoplasia 2 and 3 (CIN 2 and 3)

"Problem Pap Smear." Lastly, in many cases, we do not know why a woman's cells are demonstrating atypical changes. Fortunately, when the causes of an atypical Pap smear are benign, the abnormalities we focus on are often a one-time event and the next set of Pap smears will be normal.

When we diagnose an ASCUS on a Pap smear, we try to indicate whether in our view a reactive or a precancerous process is more likely. If your atypical Pap smear is thought to be due to reactive changes, you will see the phrase "ASCUS, favor reactive" as a diagnosis. By the same token, if your atypical Pap smear is suggestive of a precancer, it would be called "ASCUS, favor a SIL." Frequently, we are torn between whether the atypical results are seen as reflective of reactive or HPV-related changes. In those cases when we just don't know, pathologists will call a Pap smear a pure "ASCUS," which implies that

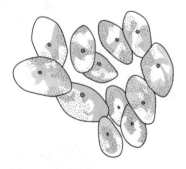
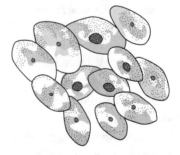

Normal
squamous cells

Atypical squamous cells of
undetermined significance
(ASCUS)

Figure 3-6. Comparison of normal squamous cells
and atypical (ASCUS) squamous cells.

it is genuinely unclear whether that which renders the cells atypical is reactive or precancerous in nature. When the diagnostician is not sure of the exact nature of the results, it is best to say so.

Subdividing ASCUS categories into "reactive," "suggestive of SIL," or just "ASCUS" is useful in predicting which women will later prove to have a SIL. In a number of studies investigating ASCUS diagnoses, including several from the Brigham and Women's Hospital in Boston and Pathology Services Inc. in Cambridge, Massachusetts, a significantly higher proportion of women with "ASCUS favor SIL" diagnoses later prove to have a SIL. This diagnosis is more serious than one which reads "ASCUS, favor reactive" or just plain "ASCUS." An even more serious diagnosis is one that reads "ASCUS, favor a high-grade SIL." A report such as this one usually triggers further clinical action (see chapter 4 for further discussions of follow-up and treatment).

SQUAMOUS INTRAEPITHELIAL LESION (SIL)

If your Pap smear report has this diagnosis, it means that you have a precancerous lesion. You have been infected with the human papillomavirus (HPV) and it has caused precancerous changes in your cervical cells resulting in a squamous intraepithelial lesion. A SIL diagnosis means the pathologist is certain about your diagnosis and that there is none of the ambiguity in your diagnosis that arises with an ASCUS diagnosis.

A SIL diagnosis on a Pap smear means the pathologist sees HPV-related cellular changes. The extent of the changes may be slight or marked. A SIL detected on a woman's cervix will be designated low-grade SIL (LSIL) if the cells show slight changes such as minimal nuclear enlargement, nuclear border irregularity and nuclear darkening (figure 3-7). A high-grade SIL (HSIL) is diagnosed if more severe changes are seen, particularly if the nucleus takes up more of the cell, for example, over 50 percent of the cell (figure 3-8).

As mentioned previously, a high-grade SIL is more worrisome than a low-grade SIL. While very much related, the two types of SIL typically differ in the type of HPV that has infected the woman (recall from chapter 1 that there are over forty different HPV subtypes that infect human genitals). Low-grade SILs reflect infection by a variety of HPV types; some, such as HPV 6 and 11, are thought to be "low-risk" for progression to cancer. Others, such as HPV

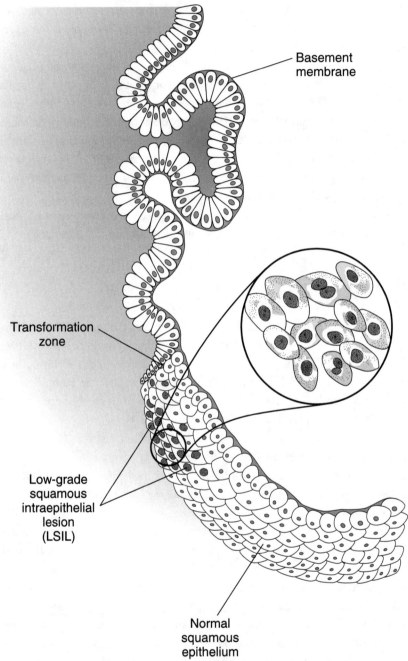

Figure 3-7. The cervical transformation zone with
low-grade squamous intraepithelial lesion (LSIL). Inset: Pap smear with LSIL cells.

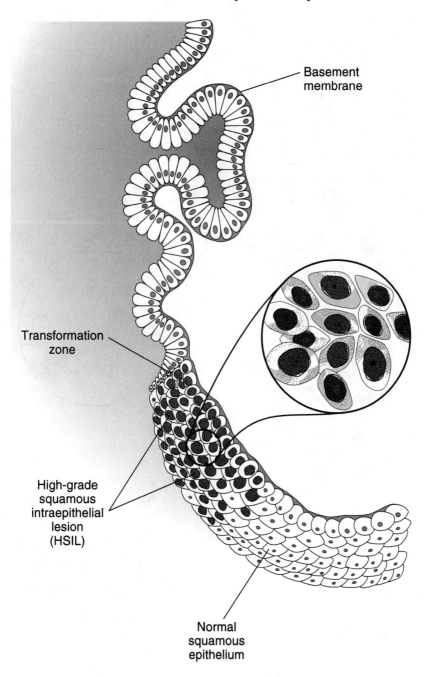

Figure 3-8. The cervical transformation zone with
high-grade squamous intraepithelial lesion (HSIL). Inset: Pap smear with HSIL cells.

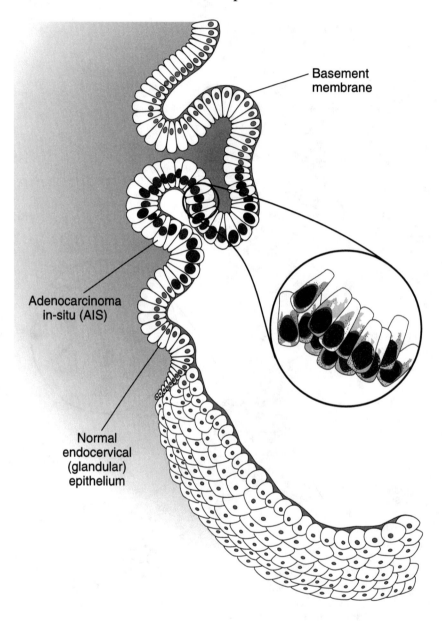

Figure 3-9. The cervical transformation zone with adenocarcinoma in-situ (AIS). Inset: Pap smear with AIS cells.

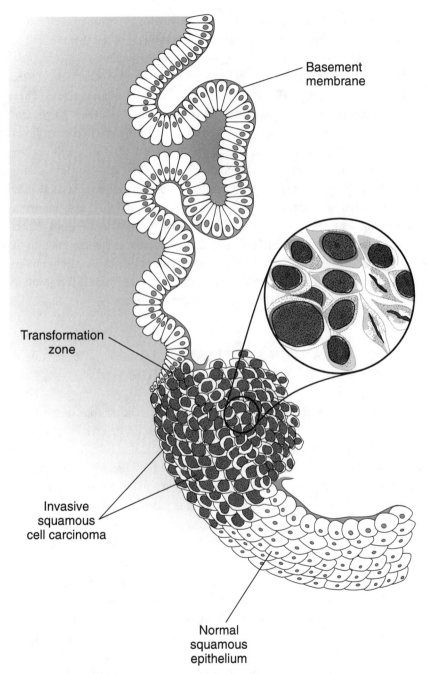

Figure 3-10. The cervical transformation zone with
invasive squamous cell carcinoma. Inset: Pap smear with squamous cell carcinoma.

16, 18, 31, and 33, are considered higher-risk viruses by virtue of their having been associated with cervical cancer cells in one study or another.

Most of these low-grade SILs (more than 50 percent) will disappear without any medical intervention. High-grade SILs, on the other hand, reflect infections by high-risk HPV types such as 16 and 18, among others. These lesions disappear on their own at a much lower rate (less than 30 percent) and, without medical treatment, may get worse and progress to cancer. Investigators estimate that anywhere from 5 to 20 percent of HSILs will develop into cancer if left untreated. High-grade SILs, in some laboratories, are further subdivided into "moderate" (Cervical intraepithelial neoplasia II [CIN II] also known as moderate dysplasia) and "severe" (CIN III also known as severe dysplasia or carcinoma-in-situ). Despite the alarming word "carcinoma," carcinoma-in-situ still refers to a precancer which is confined to the lining of the cervix and has not invaded into deeper tissues. A carcinoma-in-situ is just another name for HSIL. Most clinicians will treat HSILs similarly whether the changes are described as moderate or severe.

ATYPICAL GLANDULAR CELLS OF UNDETERMINED SIGNIFICANCE (AGUS)

Since the human papillomavirus virus targets the transition zone of the cervix and since this area consists of both squamous and endocervical (glandular) cells, it stands to reason that endocervical cells can also be affected by HPV infections. Glandular cells can also demonstrate both precancerous and cancerous changes from HPV infections although at a much decreased frequency compared with squamous cells. Why this is is currently unknown. Glandular cells can also show changes that are not diagnostic of either precancerous or reactive changes but still appear "atypical." These cases are diagnosed "atypical glandular cells of undetermined significance" or AGUS.

Like their squamous counterparts, a diagnosis of AGUS is made when the nuclei of these cells appear darker or more irregular than normally seen. The individual endocervical cells can also bunch up or appear more "crowded" on the slide. As in the case of an ASCUS diagnosis, an AGUS diagnosis can favor a reactive change or it can favor a more serious precancerous change. Again, these designations hinge on the degree of the abnormalities seen in the endocervical cells.

ADENOCARCINOMA-IN-SITU

One difference between the glandular and squamous lesions is that there are no equivalent "low-grade" lesions such as LSIL with glandular cells. The only precancerous glandular lesion has the alarming name of adenocarcinoma-in-situ or AIS. Although the word "carcinoma" is in the diagnosis, this is the glandular equivalent of a high-grade squamous intraepithelial lesion (HSIL). In this category, the cells display extreme nuclear changes of darkness and irregularity. They also display characteristic changes in the way that they appear on a slide such as crowding and piling up on each other (figure 3-9). When all of these changes can confidently be interpreted as representing a precancerous lesion, a report of adenocarcinoma-in-situ will be generated. This type of lesion is much less common than that of its squamous counterpart. Under Bethesda System guidelines, this diagnosis is categorized under the heading of "atypical glandular cells of undetermined significance" or AGUS with a strongly worded comment about the presence of adenocarcinoma-in-situ. The treatment for this lesion is also different and will be discussed in chapter 4.

ATYPICAL GLANDULAR CELLS:
ATYPICAL ENDOMETRIAL CELLS

Rarely, we will make a diagnosis on a Pap smear of atypical endometrial cells. The endometrium is the lining of the uterus, which is sloughed off monthly during the menstrual period. The endometrial cells that make up the endometrium are also a type of glandular cell with some of the same features as endocervical cells. However, unlike the endocervical cell with its tall mucus-filled cytoplasm, endometrial cells tend to be tiny and packed closely together, somewhat like grapes on a stem. The Pap smear does not sample these cells directly and was never intended as a screening method for problems in the endometrium. However, these cells can be seen on a Pap smear if it is taken during the patient's period (not a good idea, see chapter 8). Sometimes, however, it is hard to avoid a Pap smear during a woman's period due to appointment-scheduling difficulties.

From time to time, we will also see endometrial cells that look atypical, in which case they will be diagnosed as "atypical glandular cells of undetermined significance: atypical endometrial cells present." There are a number of reasons why atypical endometrial cells may end up in your Pap smear. Sometimes such cells appear "atypical" when they are really reactive or are otherwise benign. One of the more common reasons for these atypical cells includes hormone use such as hormone replacement therapy. Other causes include endometrial polyps (these are benign growths on the surface of the endometrium), leiomyomas (also known as "fibroids"), and use of an intrauterine device (IUD) for contraception. Of course, these atypical endometrial cells may also originate from either precancerous or cancerous changes in the endometrium. In the endometrium, precancerous changes are known as "endometrial hyperplasia" and the cancerous condition is called "endometrial carcinoma." A report of atypical endometrial cells will alert your clinician that your endometrium and not your cervix warrants further investigation. For more on this topic, see chapter 4.

SUSPICIOUS OR POSITIVE FOR CANCER

A Pap smear diagnosis which is "suspicious" or "positive" for cancer cells is rare. In fact such diagnoses comprise less than 1 percent of all the Pap smears we see. Keep in mind that a diagnosis of cancer means that the lesion on the cervix is no longer confined to just the lining of the cervix but has invaded through the basement membrane underlying the epithelium and into the deeper tissues with the potential to metastasize (to grow and spread). On a Pap smear, the cells show clear or diagnostic changes of malignancy or, in the case of a suspicious diagnosis, nearly diagnostic changes of malignancy.

These cancer cells are abnormal in the extreme. Squamous cancer cells can be bizarrely shaped with dark, irregular nuclei that take up almost the entire area of the cells (figure 3-10). There occasionally exists a "tumor diathesis" on the slide—a mix of blood and debris thought to derive from dead and dying tumor cells. The most common cell to become cancerous is the squamous cell leading to squamous cell carcinoma. Because these cells are less likely to be infected by HPV, endocervical or glandular cells can less commonly become malignant, producing adenocarcinomas. Rarely the cervix is host to other more unusual tumors (see chapter 6).

This diagnosis usually generates a prompt call to the clinician from the laboratory and hopefully an equally prompt call to you from your clinician.

As stomach-churning as this diagnosis may be, treatment does exist for cervical cancer, particularly when it is caught early. We will be discussing cervical cancer in detail in chapter 6.

As you saw in this chapter and in the two preceding ones, Pap smear abnormalities can be wide-ranging, encompassing changes due to infections all the way up to invasive cancer. An abnormal Pap smear will set into motion a series of clinical steps both for confirmation of a diagnosis and for treatment. Appendix A includes a list of questions you may want to ask your clinician about your Pap smear.

In the next chapter we will discuss what happens after you receive an abnormal Pap smear diagnosis. We will provide specific details on the follow-up and treatment of the abnormal Pap smear. With this information, you can proceed with any necessary treatment well-informed about what is to come. Our goal in this next chapter is to allay the fears and anxieties women commonly face when dealing with unfamiliar medical procedures.

F O U R

Follow-Up and Treatment of Abnormal Pap Smears

WHAT YOU CAN EXPECT

By now you probably have a pretty good idea of the significance of your abnormal Pap smear diagnosis. In this chapter, we will concentrate on what *follows* an abnormal Pap smear report, what kinds of further testing may be required, and which treatments you will likely undergo. As a word of caution, while we will explore the "standard" therapies for different Pap smear diagnoses, it is important to keep in mind that treatments can vary depending on your clinician's personal preferences and experience. For example, some doctors prefer to follow low-grade SILs with repeated Pap smears while others recommend more in-depth treatment.

Because we feel strongly that it is always easier to face an unknown situation when we learn through the experiences of others, we will include comments from women who have gone through various procedures for their cervical disease. We will try to answer your questions regarding discomfort during the procedures as well as what the potential is for any lasting complications. We will also cover treatments offered to women at different times in their lives, such as during pregnancy and after menopause. We hope that knowing what to expect after your abnormal Pap smear diagnosis will help to alleviate some of the anxiety that these diagnoses can cause.

REVIEW OF PAP SMEAR DIAGNOSES

This is a good time to do a quick review of possible Pap smear diagnoses. As we discussed in chapter 3, the Bethesda System of Pap smear terminology is the current convention for diagnosing the test in the United States. As also mentioned, the Bethesda System is currently undergoing changes which should be formally in place by the end of 2001.

With the current system, the terms in parentheses in the list to follow are synonyms that are still in use by some physicians and laboratories and you will occasionally see them in Pap smear or cervical biopsy reports. The Bethesda System gives us the following Pap smear diagnoses:

Within normal limits (negative)
Benign cellular changes [BCC]
Atypical squamous cells of undetermined significance [ASCUS]
Atypical glandular cells of undetermined significance [AGUS] (this category also includes adenocarcinoma-in-situ)
Low-grade squamous intraepithelial lesion [LSIL] (mild dysplasia, cervical intraepithelial neoplasia I [CIN I])
High-grade squamous intraepithelial lesion [HSIL] (moderate or severe dysplasia, cervical intraepithelial neoplasia II or III [CIN II-III], carcinoma in-situ)
Squamous cell carcinoma
Endocervical adenocarcinoma
Endometrial adenocarcinoma

Benign Cellular Changes (BCC)

Benign cellular changes refer to changes in cervical cells which deviate very slightly from normal. These changes occur mostly within a cell's nucleus and are ones that are easily recognized as benign and do not signify a SIL. Since this diagnosis is benign, it should be treated like a normal diagnosis. You do not need further follow-up and you can return for your Pap smear at the usual interval.

Atypical Squamous Cells of Undetermined Significance (ASCUS)

This diagnosis signifies that your cervix contains atypical squamous cells that the pathologist is not 100 percent sure is due to a benign process. As we mentioned in the last chapter, there are three "types" of ASCUS diagnoses: "ASCUS, favor reactive," "ASCUS, favor SIL," and just plain ASCUS. Subdividing ASCUS diagnoses gives an indication of whether the pathologist is leaning toward reactive changes or a SIL. By calling the smear ASCUS, however, she is indicating that she is not absolutely sure of the changes she is seeing. Irrespective of the exact nature of your ASCUS diagnosis you will need to have this result investigated further.

The most widely practiced follow-up for ASCUS Pap smears is simply repeating your Pap smear in three to six months. This is because a significant percentage of women with an ASCUS diagnosis will revert to normal during this time. In these cases the cell changes are probably due to a minor irritation to the cervix and not due to a SIL. A second possibility is that they were due to a SIL which has since cleared up on its own. This waiting period can seem like an eternity to a woman who has an ASCUS Pap smear result.

If you are in this situation you may wonder why you can't have your Pap smear repeated immediately. Why wait to see if anything is wrong? Couldn't cervical cancer, if present, spread during that time? These are very sensible questions. Repeating an abnormal Pap smear immediately, however, is not a good idea because your cervix needs time to recover from the trauma, however slight, of your previous Pap smear.

Your cervix undergoes a process of repair after a Pap smear which in itself can produce some atypical cells which may look enlarged and irregular. We want the repair process to complete itself before we repeat the testing. By waiting out the recommended period of time you can avoid the confusion of a Pap smear that is difficult to interpret due to the repair changes. Because of the slow-growing nature of cervical lesions, even if your ASCUS diagnosis is due to a SIL, a few months' wait is unlikely to have an effect on the severity of your eventual diagnosis. If your physician is at all concerned that you have a cancer, she will want to biopsy your cervix immediately rather than wait for the results of a repeat Pap smear. The diagnosis of an invasive cancer by cervical biopsy is not usually confused by repair changes.

If your Pap smear diagnosis was "ASCUS favor SIL," some physicians will not want simply to repeat your Pap smear in three to six months. These clinicians favor a more aggressive approach and will want to treat you as though you had received a SIL diagnosis. In that case, your follow-up will be the same as a woman with a diagnosis of LSIL, which is outlined below.

In a minority of cases, an ASCUS diagnosis will be further categorized as "ASCUS, favor HSIL" or "ASCUS, cannot rule out HSIL." These diagnoses tell the clinician that the pathologist is very concerned that the atypical cells she is seeing may be coming from an HSIL. In most instances, this diagnosis is worrisome enough that the physician will want to move quickly to make sure that you do not have an HSIL. Your physician will progress immediately to further study your cervix (see follow-up of SILs below).

If you are having a repeat Pap smear, you obviously want that second Pap smear to be of excellent quality and easily interpretable by the people who are looking at it. There are a number of steps you can take to maximize the quality of that Pap smear. We will be giving you suggestions for optimizing your Pap smear in chapter 8.

After sitting out the recommended waiting period, you should return for your repeat Pap smear. The diagnosis of this next Pap smear will determine the next course of action. The four possible diagnoses for your repeat Pap smear are: (1) negative or BCC, (2) another diagnosis of ASCUS, (3) LSIL, or (4) HSIL. While it is possible to have a repeat Pap smear that shows cervical cancer, in practice, this hardly ever happens. We discuss cervical cancer separately in chapter 6.

If your repeat Pap smear diagnosis is negative (or BCC), this is good news. It does not mean, however, that you have been given a clean bill of health. Because of the possibility that this repeat Pap smear may have missed significant cervical disease, it is recommended that you return in another three to six months for yet another Pap smear. If this third Pap smear is normal, then you can usually return to your regular yearly Pap smear and pelvic exam schedule. In general, most clinicians would like to see at least two consecutive normal Pap smears after an ASCUS Pap smear before recommending a return to an annual screening schedule.

If you receive another ASCUS on your repeat Pap smear, the time has come to move beyond sampling your cervical cells to looking more closely at your cervix. A second ASCUS diagnosis raises concerns that an undiagnosed SIL may be present. For this reason, women with two ASCUS diagnoses on their Pap smears are usually examined further with colposcopy, a diagnostic technique which we will detail below. In brief, colposcopy uses a binoculars-like magnifying instrument to look closely at the cervix. At this examination, areas that look irregular or are otherwise abnormal in appearance are biopsied. Details of cervical biopsies are covered later in this chaper.

Physicians will vary in how they approach women with ASCUS Pap smears. Some physicians are now routinely recommending HPV testing in their patients with ASCUS diagnoses. These clinicians then use the HPV test results to decide what to do next. We will discuss HPV testing in chapter 9 on new technologies. Other clinicians will not want to repeat your Pap smear but will instead move directly to colposcopy with the first atypical diagnosis. Again, your clinician will have her preferred method of following up your atypical diagnosis.

SQUAMOUS INTRAEPITHELIAL LESION (SIL)

A diagnosis of either LSIL or HSIL on a Pap smear indicates that the cells present on the Pap smear have come from a precancerous lesion, either low-grade or high-grade. Depending on your clinician, these two diagnoses may result in different treatment plans, often involving a biopsy of your cervix.

This is a good place to clarify the differences between a Pap smear and a tissue biopsy. While a Pap smear consists of a sampling of cells scraped off the surface of the cervix, a tissue biopsy is a "mini-excision" of a tiny bit of intact tissue that allows the pathologist to see a cross-section of the entire depth of the cervical lining. It is generally believed among gynecologists that a definitive diagnosis cannot be made until a biopsy has confirmed the Pap smear diagnosis. Remember that the Pap smear contains individual cells scraped off the cervix. If the cells originated in a precancerous lesion, they will have certain characteristics that allow us to diagnose them as most likely coming from a SIL. However, we cannot confirm the SIL without seeing an intact piece of tissue as a biopsy. This is analogous to finding a few bricks scattered around an empty lot. We can guess that a house most likely was once present on that lot but our suspicions are confirmed when we find intact portions of a brick wall. Tissue from a biopsy specimen is like seeing those fragments of an intact wall instead of just the bricks. We will describe the process of taking a biopsy later in this chapter.

Low-grade Squamous Intraepithelial Lesion (LSIL)

There are two ways to handle an LSIL diagnosis: (1) repeat the Pap smear in three to six months or (2) perform cervical colposcopy followed by biopsy of any visible lesions. The first option, repeating the Pap smear, may seem confusing since we have already said that we want to repeat a Pap smear that is atypical to see if it represents a SIL. Why would we then want to repeat the Pap smear yet once again when we have already identified the LSIL? Repeating the Pap smear is a viable option for LSILs because the majority of these lesions will disappear or regress on their own, thanks to the workings of a woman's immune system and the nature of HPV.

This regression may take a few years with roughly 30 percent of lesions disappearing after one year and about 60 percent after the second year. For this "watchful waiting" approach, a woman absolutely needs to be conscientious about returning for her repeat Pap smears. The purpose of these Pap smears is not only to document that the Pap smears have reverted to normal but also to make sure that there has not been progression from a low-grade lesion to a high-grade one. Remember, it is the high-grade lesions that carry the highest risk of progressing to cancer.

The exact timing of repeat Pap smears may vary depending on your clinician, but after about eighteen months of normal repeat Pap smears (generally at three- to six-month intervals), a woman can usually return to annual Pap smear screening. This plan provides time for your body's immune system to take care of the HPV infection itself without any surgical procedures. The repeat Pap smears provide reassurance that the process in your cervix is not worsening.

Some gynecologists, however, will recommend that their patients with LSIL proceed directly to colposcopy and biopsy. There is a sensible rationale behind this recommendation. We know that a significant number of women with LSIL on their Pap smears (15 to 30 percent) will later prove by biopsy to have an HSIL. How can this be? Recall that a Pap smear only provides a sampling of the very superficial cells on the top of the cervical lining. The cells from the very uppermost layer of an HSIL may be indistinguishable from those on the surface of an LSIL. The deeper layers that do not get sampled on a Pap smear, however, may demonstrate an HSIL.

As we have noted, a biopsy is required in order to make a definitive diagnosis of any cervical lesion. As an interesting note, it seems that just the act of cutting into the cervix, as with a cervical biopsy, seems to speed up the disappearance of an LSIL. It is thought that the trauma to the cervix may stimulate a woman's immune system to rid itself of the lesion at a faster rate!

High-grade Squamous Intraepithelial Lesion (HSIL)

There is little controversy surrounding the follow-up of a HSIL diagnosis on a Pap smear. These diagnoses need immediate confirmation by colposcopy and tissue biopsy and then the lesions need to be removed. Although a percentage of HSILs will spontaneously revert to normal, the number is small and there is too high of a risk that these lesions will progress to cancer if left to themselves.

Atypical Glandular Cells of Undetermined Significance (AGUS)

This diagnosis can cover a lot of ground since "atypical glandular cells" can mean either cells from the endocervical lining or from the endometrium (the lining of the uterus), since both are glandular tissues. The pathology report should make it clear what the assumed origin is for the atypical cells.

If the cells are reported as atypical glandular cells from the endometrium, your clinician may decide to perform an endometrial biopsy to make sure that you do not have any problems with your endometrium. For this biopsy, your clinician will enter your uterus through your endocervical canal using a thin instrument. Your endometrium is then gently scraped and sent to the pathology lab for examination.

Often, endometrial cells will be seen in Pap smears from women who have out-of-cycle bleeding caused by being on hormone replacement or having a known leiomyoma or "fibroid" (benign smooth muscle tumor of the uterus). In postmenopausal women, very often abnormalities of the endometrium will be heralded by abnormal bleeding. You should always see your physician to report instances of abnormal bleeding. While we do not cover problems with the endometrium in this book, there are other sources of information about the endometrium outlined in Appendix B.

If the cells are reported as atypical glandular cells from the endocervix, then the concern is that you have an adenocarcinoma-in-situ (AIS) as we discussed in the last chapter. As with ASCUS diagnoses, your AGUS report may favor reactive changes; it may favor AIS; or it may remain unspecified. Under the idiosyncrasies of the Bethesda System, a diagnosis of AIS will still be diagnosed as AGUS with a strongly worded comment about the presence of AIS. A diagnosis of "AGUS, favor reactive endocervical cells" can probably be handled in the same way as a reactive ASCUS diagnosis, that is by repeat Pap smears. A diagnosis of "AGUS, favor AIS" on the other hand, is a more serious diagnosis and requires colposcopy and biopsies with endocervical curettage described later in this chapter. Because glandular lesions can hide deep in the endocervical canal, if the biopsies are negative and either repeat Pap smears or a review of your current Pap smear still looks like AIS, you will most likely need a cone biopsy, details of which are provided later in this chapter. This procedure is done to make sure you do not have adenocarcinoma-in-situ. An AGUS lesion that is not otherwise specified will also often lead to colposcopy, endocervical curettage, sometimes cervical biopsies, and occasionally endometrial sampling to ensure the atypical glandular cells aren't arising from the endometrium.

Squamous Cell Carcinoma and Adenocarcinoma

The important topic of cervical cancer, both squamous cell cancer and adenocarcinoma, are handled separately in chapter 6. The topic of endometrial carcinoma is not discussed in this book. We offer resources for learning about this malignancy in Appendix B.

PROCEDURES FOR DIAGNOSING AND TREATING PRECANCEROUS LESIONS

We now move on to more detailed descriptions of the various procedures we have been outlining. Except for the cone biopsy, these can all take place in your physician's office. They can also be performed by a licensed and experienced nurse practitioner. The diagnostic and tissue sampling methods are listed below:

Cervical colposcopy
Cervical biopsy
Endocervical curettage

Cryotherapy

Loop Procedure, also known as Loop Electrosurgical Excision Procedure (LEEP®)

Cone biopsy ("cold knife cone")

Cervical Colposcopy

Cervical colposcopy is a special procedure that involves closely examining your cervix with special binoculars that magnify your cervical tissue like a microscope. This inspection allows recognition of subtle changes signifying the presence of abnormalities such as SILs. These areas can then be biopsied using special instruments. If your Pap smears are performed by a primary-care doctor untrained in colposcopy, he or she probably will not do this examination. Instead, you will receive an appointment with another physician or nurse practitioner who is experienced in the technique.

For your colposcopy, you will be in the same lithotomy position as you are for your annual Pap smear and pelvic examination. Just as with your pelvic examination, a speculum will be inserted into your vagina, holding apart your vaginal tissues so that your cervix is clearly visible.

The colposcope looks similar to a pair of binoculars and is mounted on a movable and adjustable stand that is placed between your legs. The goal of colposcopy is to inspect your cervix closely, especially the transformation zone area where cervical precancers typically start. The colposcope magnifies your cervix between three and ten times.

To further highlight any abnormal areas, the surface of your cervix is washed with a 2 to 5 percent acetic acid solution, which is essentially a dilute solution of vinegar. The acetic acid serves to dry out your cervical cells which helps in the recognition of abnormal areas. As an additional step, a different solution called Lugol's solution may be applied to your cervix. Lugol's solution is iodine-based and stains your cervix yellow. Any areas of your cervix with precancerous changes will stand out since they remain unstained in contrast to the surrounding yellow-stained normal tissue. A special filter on the colposcope also serves to highlight the blood vessels of your cervix. Abnormalities in the appearance of these vessels can also help to identify a SIL. The process of examining your cervix takes about ten minutes.

What do abnormal areas of your cervix look like? A normal cervix looks like a very smooth, glistening, firm, tan-pink doughnut (figure 4-1). Using

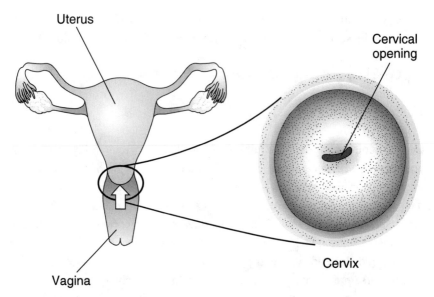

Figure 4-1. The cervix as seen during a pelvic examination and colposcopy.

the colposcope with magnification, filters, and special solutions, abnormal areas may appear paler, more irregular, or roughened compared with the surrounding normal tissue. The normal surface of the cervix has almost no blood vessels and an increase in their number and prominence suggests the presence of a SIL.

During your colposcopy, your clinician will typically draw a doughnut-shaped picture of your cervix on your medical chart denoting the location, size, and shape of any abnormal areas. The convention for identifying location on the cervix is as if looking at the face of a clock with 12 o'clock straight up and 6 o'clock straight down and the other positions proceeding around the clock face. If an abnormal area is identified on your cervix, your physician may note, for example, "an irregular pale area with abnormal blood vessels at 2 o'clock."

As part of inspecting the transformation zone, your clinician will look with the colposcope as high into your endocervical canal as possible. The entire transformation zone must be seen in a successful colposcopic examination. This is to ensure that no abnormalities are lurking in this area. In some women, particularly older women after menopause, the opening to the endocervical canal can be quite small and tight, a condition known as "cervical stenosis." In such cases, a special instrument called an endocervical

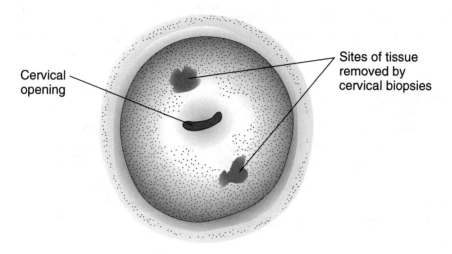

Cervical opening

Sites of tissue removed by cervical biopsies

Figure 4-2. The cervix after cervical biopsies.

speculum may be used to open up the cervix so that this area can be inspected more thoroughly.

Other situations where colposcopy can be difficult are obesity and vaginal atrophy. Colposcopy in obese women may be difficult simply due to the additional mass of tissue that collapses the vagina and prevents clear visualization of the cervix. "Vaginal atrophy" refers to a woman's vagina becoming somewhat contracted and tightened after menopause. This can make even inserting a speculum a challenge, much less visualizing a woman's cervix. This atrophic condition can be improved with use of a vaginal estrogen cream applied for a month prior to colposcopy.

Cervical Biopsy

A biopsy of the cervix may be performed during colposcopy if your clinician has identified abnormal areas. The goal of cervical biopsies is to cut out small pieces of your cervix to examine under the microscope so that a diagnosis can be rendered. Biopsies generally do not serve to completely remove a SIL. Unlike a Pap smear, cervical biopsies give us a look at intact cervical tissue from top to bottom so that all the well-described features of a SIL, if present, can be fully evaluated.

For women with abnormal areas identified by colposcopy, "directed" biopsies will be taken specifically targeting the abnormal areas. Occasionally, random biopsies may be taken if no abnormalities are noted by colposcopy but your clinician is nonetheless suspicious of a SIL. The instruments for cervical biopsies are long-handled pinchers with small sharp teeth for getting a grip on the smooth surface of your cervix. The biopsy instruments will take a bite out of your cervix with the biopsy dimensions measuring about one-eighth-inch square. Anywhere from one to several biopsies may be taken depending on what is seen with colposcopy (figure 4-2). Each biopsy takes only a few seconds to obtain and is placed into plastic containers with formalin fixative labeled with your name. These are sent to the pathology laboratory for processing and microscopic inspection by pathologists.

Endocervical Curettage

Many women who undergo colposcopy will have a special type of biopsy taken called an "endocervical curettage." This will generally be done even if they have no other biopsies of their cervix taken. The endocervical canal is the tiny tunnel leading up from your cervix into your uterus. Colposcopy can inspect only the very opening of this canal and the canal's upper reaches are essentially a blind area of your cervix. Gynecologists worry about SILs hiding high up in the canal where they can't easily be detected. To address this concern, an endocervical curettage allows your physician to scrape tissue from the canal and have that tissue looked at under a microscope.

"Curettage" is a French word which means "to scrape" and that pretty much sums up this procedure. Using a long-handled instrument with a small spoon-shaped open centered end called a "curet," your physician will reach up into your endocervical canal and scrape along the sides to collect this tissue in a container. This process takes about 30 to 45 seconds to complete and is usually done after any biopsies are taken. The tissue obtained will also be sent to the pathology laboratory for processing and inspection by a pathologist. Some older women with very narrow endocervical canals may need the canal first slightly stretched or dilated with an endocervical speculum in order to get an endocervical sample.

WHAT CAN YOU EXPECT TO FEEL DURING AND AFTER YOUR COLPOSCOPY, CERVICAL BIOPSY, AND ENDOCERVICAL CURETTAGE?

What do women experience during a colposcopy procedure that includes cervical biopsies and endocervical curettage? The sensations experienced by women vary. A mild burning sensation is felt by some women when the acetic acid is applied to their cervix. Other women describe a cold sensation from the acetic acid. Some women experience minimal discomfort other than a tugging sensation when the biopsy is taken.

Other women, however, report a sharp pinching sensation with biopsies. One woman we spoke to likened the feeling to "pain at my very core." She did acknowledge, however, that she was deeply modest and the whole procedure was very upsetting to her. Another woman said that colposcopies and biopsies were "a piece of cake" since her physician applied a local anesthetic prior to taking the biopsies. She said that she had had biopsies both with and without local anesthesia and the anesthetic made "all the difference in the world."

Another woman we spoke with strongly suggested taking over-the-counter pain relievers such as Tylenol or Ibuprofen an hour or so prior to the procedure. She neglected to do this before her first set of biopsies and these she stated were "excruciating." Having a little pain relief on board for her second set of biopsies made them more tolerable. For other women, meditative breathing techniques such as those learned in yoga or even Lamaze breathing learned for labor helped them during the actual procedures.

According to Dr. Diane McGrory, a gynecologist in practice at Gynecology Partners out of Newton-Wellesley Hospital in Massachusetts, "residents [physicians in training] are told that there are no pain fibers on the cervix, which I do not agree with. Residents are taught that you can burn, clamp, freeze, and biopsy the cervix without anesthesia. Most dentists would not do a biopsy on the oral mucous membranes without an anesthetic. Gynecologists in general do not anesthetize the cervix prior to biopsy because they were not trained to do so." Dr. McGrory uses 1 percent xylocaine® without epinepherine or a small amount of 2 percent xylocaine® jelly prior to cervical biopsies. She feels that her patients are more comfortable with this procedure. Dr. McGrory states: "I think women need to ask for local anesthesia."

Several women stated that a big problem for them was that they were not *forewarned* that their physicians were planning colposcopy and biopsy when they came for their follow-up appointments after an abnormal Pap smear. One woman said that hearing her physician say the word "biopsy" shocked her since she only had heard the word used in the context of cancer. Her biopsies were deeply painful, she suspects, because she felt out-of-control and the procedures were unexpected.

If you have been called back to your physician's office for follow-up of an abnormal Pap smear, you may want to quiz your doctor or the office staff about what you should expect at this follow-up appointment. Is it merely for a repeat Pap smear? Is the clinician planning to do colposcopy and biopsies? Is it all right if you take some Ibuprofen prior to the procedure? You will not want to take aspirin since this drug may prolong bleeding. If the receptionist or office nurse is not sure, leave a message for your clinician to call you with answers to these questions. Perhaps the nurse can get the answers and then call you back. We have heard repeatedly from women that the sensation of being *out-of-control* and not knowing what to expect magnifies their anxieties and probably their pain perceptions in these procedures.

Endocervical curettage typically produces a strong cramping sensation lasting the length of the procedure, about 30 to 45 seconds. Once again, "premedicating" before your procedure with an over-the-counter medication that you might use for menstrual cramps such as Ibuprofen or Tylenol® may reduce this discomfort.

The primary side effects of these procedures are lower abdominal pain and bleeding. Any bleeding from your cervix at the biopsy site can largely be controlled at the time of the biopsies. Your physician will take steps to minimize bleeding by taking as few biopsies as necessary and having on hand materials to limit bleeding. They may use sterile gauze for packing the biopsy sites which helps your blood to clot. Your physician may use Monsel's paste (a dark iron-containing mixture) to stop the bleeding. If a large amount of bleeding occurs, electric cautery tools may be used to close off the end of bleeding vessels. This serves to immediately plug the small bleeding vessels and slow down bleeding.

All these steps serve to reduce the amount of bleeding you may experience after the procedure is finished. After your colposcopy you may experience light spotting for a few days to a week. Your spotting may be of a dark brown color due to the different colored solutions used during the colposcopy. The discharge may also feel a little gritty if Monsel's paste was used. The bleeding should not be any heavier than your menstrual flow. Any prolonged or heavy bleeding should be reported at once to your physician who will want to examine you to see what is producing the bleeding.

As with any biopsy elsewhere in your body, there is a small risk of infection but this is a very rare occurrence. The human body is perfectly capable of quickly healing the small areas from biopsies and there is no need for antibiotics to be given after this procedure. If women experience a fever or a marked increase in pelvic pain after these procedures they should contact their physician at once.

Pain and discomfort after cervical biopsies are usually not a problem but if it arises, over-the-counter medications such as Tylenol® or Ibuprofen should help. As mentioned, aspirin should be avoided after procedures where bleeding is produced because aspirin itself can increase bleeding. A hot pad placed on the lower abdomen may be of help with any pain or discomfort. To prevent further bleeding or infection it is recommended that women abstain from sexual intercourse for two to three weeks after the procedure. It is also recommended that they do not use tampons or douche during that time. It will take about three to four weeks for the cervix to heal. Patients we have spoken with emphasized that women will want to treat themselves gently the day of their biopsies. They may want to take the day off from work and do whatever comforts them the most, whether it be lying down with a book or having a trusted friend come over.

AFTER COLPOSCOPY: YOUR CERVICAL BIOPSY AND ENDOCERVICAL CURETTAGE PATHOLOGY REPORT

After the colposcopy, you should ask your physician what she saw. Did she see any areas that looked suspicious for precancerous changes? Did she take any cervical biopsies or perform an endocervical curettage? Was she able to see your transformation zone, the most likely area for precancers? Appendix A contains a number of questions you may want to ask your clinician pertaining to your colposcopy.

Whatever information you glean from your physician, keep in mind that whatever she saw using the colposcope needs to be confirmed by the pathologist who reviews the cervical biopsy. Things other than SILs can change the appearance of your cervix, so while it may appear abnormal during colposcopy, the biopsy results may not indicate precancerous changes. Inflammation of your cervix, for example, is notorious for producing the appearance of a SIL by colposcopy. In other words, the true answer about any cervical disease will be in the pathology results for your cervical biopsy and endocervical curettage.

It will be several days after your colposcopy procedure before you can receive news of your cervical biopsies and endocervical curettage. The laboratory will provide these results to your physician. If a precancer is found on any of your biopsy specimens, it will probably be indicated as either a low-grade or high-grade squamous intraepithelial lesion (LSIL or HSIL). Some laboratories use the standard Bethesda System for their Pap smear diagnoses and other terminology for their cervical biopsies. Other language you may see is "mild dysplasia" or "slight dysplasia" which has the same meaning as LSIL. Similarly, "moderate dysplasia" or "severe dysplasia" has the same meaning as HSIL. These diagnoses confirm that you have an infection by human papillomavirus (HPV) that is producing precancerous changes in your cervix.

In many instances, no precancerous changes are found on a woman's cervical biopsies. Very commonly these biopsies will show the effects of inflammation on the cervix. The diagnosis in such cases will indicate a cervicitis (meaning "inflammation of the cervix"). Since the cervical tissues are "reacting" to the inflammation, the reports may state the presence of "reactive atypia" which is not a precancer. Reactive atypia is seen when cells in the epithelium appear slightly enlarged and more irregular than normal.

If your biopsies have not revealed a SIL, an important comment to look for in your pathology report is the *absence* of your cervical transformation zone. It is from this area that biopsies are usually taken and which have the greatest likelihood of revealing dysplasia. If your pathology report says the transformation or "transition" zone is not present, this means your biopsy was taken from a less than ideal place. If this is the case, you may want to ask your physician his reasons for selecting these sites for a biopsy. Perhaps this was the only area that had any hint of abnormality. Confirm with him that your transformation zone was well seen and well inspected for abnormalities.

The pathology report for your endocervical curettage should be looked at for some key features. The presence of SIL on a curettage indicates that a SIL is present high in the endocervical canal. If your diagnosis is HSIL, this may mean you will need to have more extensive surgery to completely remove the lesion. Also check your curettage report to see if the sample was considered to be ample enough for evaluation by the pathologists. Endocervical curettages are notorious for being very skimpy in quantity, with too little endocervical tissue for an accurate diagnosis for the presence or absence of dysplasia. If your report says that your specimen contained too little tissue for diagnosis, your clinician may want to repeat the curettage.

WHEN YOUR PAP SMEAR
AND BIOPSY REPORTS DON'T AGREE

The ideal situation is to have all of a woman's results agree. It is helpful if the results from her Pap smear, her colposcopy, and her cervical biopsy all show the same findings thus allowing her physician to confidently plan how next to treat the SIL. A confusing situation arises when there is disagreement between these results. We discuss this situation in the next chapter on the "Problem Pap Smear."

Cervical Laser and Cryotherapy

There are several methods available to remove a SIL. Two of these methods are cryotherapy (a freezing technique) or carbon dioxide laser therapy. Both of these can be used after your SIL Pap smear diagnosis has been confirmed by a cervical biopsy. Both laser and cryotherapy can be done in your doctor's office although sometimes laser therapy will be done in an operating room using general anesthesia. Both of these procedures are very effective in removing SILs, both LSIL and HSIL, providing the entire SIL can be seen.

A big disadvantage of both laser and cryotherapy are that while these therapies might efficiently remove cervical lesions, they also destroy them so completely that there is no tissue left for a pathologist to examine using a microscope. Microscopic examination is important in these lesions because we want to verify and document the severity of an HPV lesion and to tell if it is completely excised. Since no cervical tissue fragment is actually removed during laser or cryotherapy, there is no tissue for a pathologist to examine for a diagnosis. With these therapies there is always a chance that a woman may have an invasive cancer rather than a precancer and that invasive cancer could go undiagnosed. For this reason, many physicians would prefer to do other surgical procedures to remove a SIL, such as a loop, described later in this chapter. These procedures provide tissue for a pathologist to examine with a microscope.

Cryotherapy utilizes an extremely cold metal instrument, cooled using chemical refrigerants, to freeze the areas of your cervix that the colposcopy showed to be abnormal. The process typically takes about three to five minutes. As mentioned, no tissue is taken for examination under the microscope by pathology.

What can you expect to feel during cryotherapy? Many women feel cramping, sometimes severe, and a stinging sensation during the freezing process. Afterwards, you may feel continued discomfort as a dull pain for which you can take Ibuprofen four times a day for several days. Warm tub soaks twice a day are also recommended to alleviate this discomfort. Women also may have a clear yellow discharge for a few weeks as their cervix heals over the period of a month. As with the other cervical procedures we've discussed, it is recommended that you abstain from intercourse for the two or three weeks after your cryotherapy.

Cervical Loop

If you have an HSIL identified on your cervical biopsies, the next step taken is surgical removal of the lesion by a method that produces tissue for examination by pathologists. The current method of achieving this goal is by the loop procedure. This is also known by the name Loop Electrosurgical Excision procedure or LEEP® for short, a procedure that has been in use in the United States since the late 1980s. For most women a loop can be performed in their doctor's office. About 25 percent of women, however, need to have their loop in the operating room for various reasons. For example, women who are very anxious or have a low threshold for pain may need general anesthesia in an operating room as may women whose cervix is difficult to visualize.

With a loop, a woman is given the opportunity for treatment and a microscopic diagnosis at the same time. Loop instruments are slender pencil-like instruments outfitted with a fine wire loop at one end. The entire instrument is electrically charged, heating the fine wire loop and making it capable of cutting tissue as neatly as a very sharp scalpel. The wire loop sizes are usually three-quarters-inch wide, although more narrow wires may be used in certain situations. Another electrically charged pencil-like instrument used during a loop has a small round quarter-inch ball at one end. This instrument is used for controlling bleeding. Both of these instruments are connected by wiring to an electrical source controlled by foot switches.

If you are having a loop, you will again be positioned in that same on-your-back, knees-up-and-to-the-side lithotomy position. This time, however, your physician will be using instruments that carry electrical currents and care will be taken to use insulated speculums and instruments to pull aside your vaginal tissues. Since the electric current running through the loop instruments will essentially burn through cervical tissues to provide a sample, a built-in smoke evacuator helps your physician clearly see what she is cutting.

As was done at your first colposcopy, your cervix will be painted with acetic acid and possibly Lugol's solution to better visualize any HPV lesions. This time you will receive a local anesthetic in the form of lidocaine (identical to the numbing medicine xylocaine® as is used for dental procedures). This local anesthesia has an extra ingredient, epinephrine, which acts to reduce bleeding. This will be given as four equally spaced injections either all around your cervix or just around the identified lesion. This type of cervical anesthesia is known as a "paracervical block."

After the anesthetic has taken effect, the lesion will be removed using a slow and steady swipe of the wire loop, which typically goes to a tissue depth of about a quarter inch (figure 4-3). The removed tissue is then sent to the pathology laboratory for diagnosis. Depending on the size of a woman's lesion, more tissue may need to be removed. After removal, there will be a raw area on the surface of the cervix. This surface will be examined using a colposcope and if any residual lesion is present, it, too, will be excised. An endocervical curettage is then performed to sample the endocervical canal for disease. Next, any bleeding vessels in the raw surface will be electrically burned and closed off with the ball-tipped instrument. As a final step, this area is packed with the blood-stopping Monsel's paste which adheres to the walls of the raw surface. The process typically takes about five to ten minutes although you can expect to be on the table somewhat longer.

WHAT YOU MIGHT EXPERIENCE
DURING AND AFTER YOUR LOOP

If adequate anesthesia is given, most women do not feel much during the procedure itself, other than dull tugging sensations on their cervixes. Women may feel the lidocaine injections as deep dull pain sometimes with cramping. Again, deep breathing techniques may be useful as this is being done.

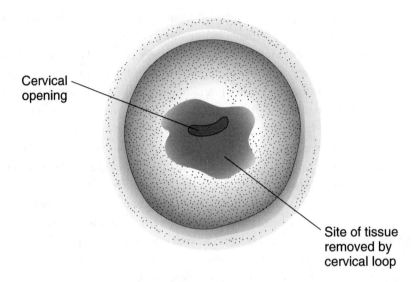

Figure 4-3. The cervix after a loop.

Women can also sometimes experience their heart racing from the lidocaine. The endocervical curettage often produces cramping while the canal is being scraped. Women describe the entire procedure as somewhat noisy due to the smoke evacuator.

As with cervical biopsies and endocervical curettage, most of the after-effects revolve around pain and bleeding. Women may experience dull painful sensations in their lower abdomen for a few days after the procedure, beginning the first day as the local anesthetic wears off. Again, the subjective descriptions of pain vary among individuals. Some women require several days in bed with over-the-counter medications. Others are up and about quickly. If the pain appears to worsen a few days after the procedure, you should alert your physician. It may indicate a complication from the procedure such as an infection. For the majority of women, a dark brown vaginal discharge due to Monsel's paste is noted after a loop. This may continue for a few weeks after the procedure.

As with the other procedures described in this chapter, to limit your risk of infection and bleeding you should abstain from sexual intercourse, tampon use, or douching for two or three weeks after your procedure. In addition, after a loop, you should not engage in heavy lifting or aerobic exercise for seven to ten days. Full healing of your cervix will take about six weeks.

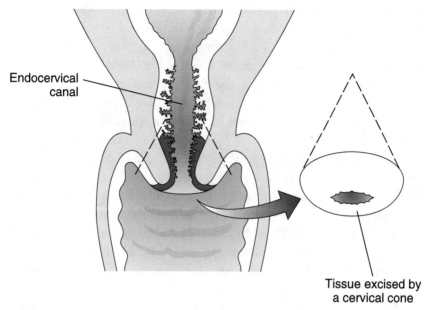

Endocervical
canal

Tissue excised by
a cervical cone

Figure 4-4. Cone-shaped tissue removed from the cervix during a cone procedure.

Cervical Conization

A cervical cone is a different and more extensive surgical procedure and is another possible treatment for your SIL. This is performed in the operating room using either local, spinal, or general anesthesia and involves greater cost and risk. A cone is reserved for women who have cervical biopsies that indicate a concern about invasive cancer rather than a precancerous lesion limited to the lining of the cervix. Women who have high-grade SILs extending high into their endocervical canals may be candidates for a cone. It is also typically used on women with a diagnosis of endocervical adeno-carcinoma-in-situ. This procedure removes a larger and deeper amount of cervical tissue than a loop.

A cervical cone is performed using a sharp surgical scalpel and typically cuts deeper into a woman's cervical tissues than a loop (figure 4-4). There are also some new linear wire electrode devices available for excising a cervical cone that yield similar results to scalpel excision with less trauma. The incision cuts completely around the cervix and will require suturing or sewing of a cervix after the cone tissue is removed. The tissue produced from this deeper cutting is an elongated doughnutlike cone which should be deep enough to get around any minimally invasive tumor, if present. This is not the recommended procedure for women who obviously have deeply invasive tumors. Treatment of invasive tumors is covered in chapter 6.

Since this operation is more involved and removes a good portion of tissue, you should expect to have a longer "downtime." Some physicians suggest that you may have a quicker recovery by optimizing your diet and engaging in moderate amounts of exercise prior to your surgery. After the procedure, some women have problems with pain that lasts a number of days. One woman recommended that patients take the full course of pain medication prescribed. She stated that although she usually does not like to take any medications in her everyday life, in this instance, she allowed herself a full measure of pain relief. Again, expect a significant amount of time during which you may be confined to bed or at least will not be doing anything too strenuous. Again, abstinence from sexual intercourse, tampon use, or douching is recommended for two to three weeks. Most women need a good one to two weeks of recovery time. This will be a time for dipping into your support systems whether they be partners, spouses, sisters, or friends. A surprising number of women relied on their mothers to provide comfort at this time.

POSSIBLE COMPLICATIONS OF LOOP AND CONIZATION

The main complications of the loop and conization methods are bleeding, cervical infection, cervical stenosis (marked narrowing of the cervix), and problems with infertility and pregnancy.

Excessive bleeding during and after the procedure can occur for several reasons. Some women have problems with slow blood clotting causing problems during and after a loop or conization. If you know that you have such a problem, be sure to inform your clinician prior to the procedure. Bleeding can also occur if the loop is not performed properly. One such mishap is when the electrically charged hot wire is placed in the wrong area and cuts through a large cervical artery. Another consequence of a loop is allowing the cutting wire to inadvertently come in contact with a woman's vagina and produce cuts that cause bleeding. These instances of bleeding need to be controlled at the time of the procedure usually with the help of electrical devices that burn the ends of bleeding vessels.

A few women (around 1 to 2 percent) may experience bleeding after a loop or conization which requires a physician's attention. Often a single vessel oozing blood may be found in the loop's raw surface (the area remaining after the tissue has been cut away). This will be burned again by the electric ball and Monsel's paste will be reapplied. It is recommended that you do not engage in heavy lifting or aerobic exercise for seven to ten days after a loop or cone biopsy. The highest risk for bleeding after these procedures is seven days.

Infection occurring after loop or conization is an uncommon complication. In some instances it is thought to represent worsening of an untreated infection that a woman had prior to her surgery. The presence of fevers, chills, and prolonged pain suggests this rare complication and should prompt a call to your clinician.

These procedures, by removing the outermost portion of your cervix, act to alter the shape of the cervix and may rarely lead to cervical scarring or cervical stenosis. Cones are probably the worst offenders due to the larger amount of tissue taken; however, laser, cryotherapy, and the loop technique can also carry this complication. With cervical stenosis, a woman's endocervical canal can be scarred to such a degree that it's just a tiny opening, or it could even close up altogether. Resulting problems include blocked menstrual flow, painful menstruation, and infertility. For women in their childbearing years, cervical stenosis may result in sperm not being able to pass through the canal to allow pregnancy. There are options for women if this complication occurs. Intrauterine insemination can bypass a stenotic cervix so that pregnancy can occur. Older women in their menopausal years appear to be at particularly high risk for cervical stenosis. This could prevent their endocervical canal from being examined in the future. Cervical stenosis can be reversed using special instruments to reopen a woman's cervix. Adhering to your doctor's recommendations for follow-up after your surgery is important, since the earlier cervical stenosis is detected and treated, the better the outcome will be.

There is also a risk of these procedures weakening the cervix so that it does not function properly to keep a pregnancy inside the uterus. Women with this uncommonly occurring problem, called an "incompetent cervix," are at risk for miscarrying their pregnancies, premature delivery of their babies, and even low-birth-weight babies. If this problem occurs, it can be remedied by actually sewing closed the cervical opening once a woman becomes pregnant. This procedure is known as "cervical cerclage."

WHO SHOULD NOT UNDERGO A LOOP OR CONIZATION

The vast majority of women with diagnoses of cervical precancers can safely and successfully undergo loops. There are a few women, however, for whom the procedure is not advised. Pregnant women should not undergo these procedures due to the risk to the fetus. Women with bleeding problems who are at risk for bleeding complications need to inform their clinicians of their conditions. Lastly, women who have an obvious invasive cervical cancer should not have a loop or cone biopsy. These women need different procedures (see chapter 6).

YOUR LOOP OR CONE PATHOLOGY REPORT

The same terms that are used in diagnosing a SIL on a biopsy are employed on your loop or cone: LSIL (mild or slight dysplasia) or HSIL (moderate to severe dysplasia). An additional feature of the loop report, not available from other reports, is the status of the edges or margins of your specimen. In other words, examination of the edges of your specimen will tell you if your clinician re-moved the entire SIL or if some was left behind. If the edges of the tissue show SIL, then we know the SIL was cut through and some SIL may still remain in the woman. If the edges show normal tissue without SIL, we surmise the SIL was completely removed. Loop reports should always say if a lesion was com-pletely removed. There are times, however, when it is difficult to be sure about this, usually because of tissue irregularities or the effects of the electrical cut-ting (cautery) on a loop specimen's tissues. In such instances the pathology report may state that the edges or margins are inconclusive or indeterminate.

Your loop report will also include a report on your endocervical curet-tage. The presence of residual SIL on an endocervical curettage indicates dis-ease high in the endocervical canal. Since the endocervical curettage is per-formed after the loop, this result means the SIL was incompletely removed and is still present higher in the endocervical canal. In this case a woman may need yet another loop.

Not uncommonly, a woman's loop report will not reveal any evidence of a remaining SIL. In these instances, we can surmise that the lesion was com-pletely removed at the time of the initial cervical biopsy leaving no residual precancerous changes. In addition, a woman's immune system may have helped eliminate the lesion. The absence of a SIL on a loop report does not mean you had a loop for no reason. The loop itself is necessary for reassuring you that your SIL was completely removed. Appendix A offers questions for your clinician about your loop or cone.

HOW SUCCESSFUL ARE THESE TREATMENTS AT CURING PRECANCEROUS LESIONS?

All of the procedures we have described in this chapter have about the same success rate of eliminating SILs from your cervix. They all are about 85 to 95 percent successful. The vast majority of women will have normal Pap smears after their procedures, provided their lesions were completely excised. Some woman may need their lesions treated more than once for a complete removal. How do we know if a lesion is completely excised? Having a loop or cone is really the only way to be certain as it is the only procedure that will yield tissue that can be properly evaluated at its edges or margins. Treatment by laser or cryotherapy will not tell you whether your lesion has been completely removed.

It is critical to remember that successful elimination of your SIL is not the same thing as being cured of your HPV infection. Your SIL may be gone but HPV may still be lurking in your adjacent normal-appearing tissue. Approximately 20 percent of women will test positive for HPV after removal of their SIL. The likelihood is high, however, that your body will rid itself of any residual HPV. As was mentioned earlier, the actual physical trauma of surgical removal of SILs appears to stimulate an immune response which serves to eliminate most residual SILs. Keep in mind that you may be reinfected with HPV in the future although it is unlikely that you will be reinfected with the same virus from your current partner since you are now likely "immune" to that particular HPV subtype or subtypes. Since so many issues surrounding reinfection and viral latency are unknown, it is critical to continue having Pap smears to check for recurrent SILs.

LONG-TERM FOLLOW-UP AFTER YOUR LOOP OR CONE

If your loop or cone was successful at completely removing your SIL, the next step is to ensure that this is really the case. This follow-up is done with

Pap smears. It is recommended that after a loop, a woman have repeat Pap smears every three to six months. If these Pap smears are normal for three consecutive visits, she can return to once-a-year screening.

If your loop or cone did not completely remove the lesion, especially if your endocervical curettage shows precancerous changes, your clinician may elect to remove even more tissue. This may be done by performing yet another loop, one that takes tissue from higher up in the endocervical canal.

HYSTERECTOMY FOR TREATMENT OF PRECANCERS

Hysterectomy or removal of the uterus as a treatment of SILs is very rarely recommended or performed. In some instances a high-grade SIL may not be able to be completely removed by loop or conization and a woman will need more extensive surgery. This is necessary in only 5 to 10 percent of women with SIL. It would be inappropriate to perform a hysterectomy for a low-grade lesion, which has such a high chance of disappearing on its own and a low risk of developing into cervical cancer. If a woman with a high-grade SIL is difficult to treat by the loop or cone methods and is past wanting to become pregnant, a hysterectomy may be performed. Some women may also have coexisting gynecologic conditions treatable by hysterectomy which push both her and her doctor toward removing her uterus. Such other conditions include dysfunctional uterine bleeding (noncancerous bleeding seen in women in the years around menopause), uterine fibroids, or uterine prolapse (a dropping down of the uterus into the vagina due to the weakening of uterine support tissues which occurs with age). With a hysterectomy, the entire uterus with cervix is removed while a woman is in an operating room and under general anesthesia. What women experience after this operation is discussed in chapter 6 in the section describing hysterectomy as a treatment for cervical cancer.

Having a hysterectomy for treatment of a high-grade SIL should not be taken as the ultimate cure for precancerous lesions. Although you won't have to worry about cervical cancer anymore, a small number of women (1 to 7 percent) will have HPV-related precancers show up in their vagina or vulva after their hysterectomies for HSIL. Lesions in these regions have different names, vaginal intraepithelial neoplasia or VAIN in the vagina and vulvar intraepithelial neoplasia or VIN in the vulva. As in the cervix, these lesions can be either low-grade or high-grade with a low or high probability of progressing to cancer in those areas. It is important for women after hysterectomies for SILs to continue having Pap smears and pelvic examinations to look for the presence of any HPV-related lesions in the vagina or vulvar tissues. These lesions can also progress to cancer of the vagina or vulva.

ALTERNATIVE TREATMENT OF CERVICAL PRECANCERS

The above treatment guidelines are needed to rid your cervix of a precancerous lesion. No other treatments have been shown to effectively remove a SIL. There is plenty of room, however, for lifestyle changes that may improve the effectiveness of your immune system. Nutrition, stress reduction, and changes in a woman's sexual habits can all come into play. These will be discussed in further detail in chapter 10.

In the next chapter we will discuss specific situations that can pose difficulties in interpreting your Pap smear. Some of these situations occur at somewhat predictable times in a woman's life. Other situations are more difficult to identify and may result in problems in Pap smear interpretation.

F I V E

The Problem Pap Smear

If you received an ASCUS diagnosis this year, you were one of an estimated two to three million women in America with an atypical Pap smear. Unlike Pap smears that contain a SIL, your Pap smear occupies that uncomfortable zone between clearly normal and clearly abnormal. There is no definitive proof that you have a cervical precancer, yet you have not been given a clean bill of health.

For most women, a repeat Pap smear will clear up this ambiguous situation. Usually, either the second Pap smear will show a normal status or it will demonstrate a clear-cut HPV-related lesion. However, for an unfortunate minority of women, this does not happen. These women receive ASCUS diagnoses repeatedly. They undergo colposcopies, sometimes multiple times, as well as biopsies, without a cervical precancer ever being documented.

Jeannie is a sophomore in college with jet-black hair and blue eyes. She has had four atypical Pap smears in the past year and a half along with three sets of biopsies. All of her biopsies were called "normal." She is beyond frustrated. Her numerous doctor's appointments disrupt her busy schedule of work and school. After her biopsies, she cannot have sex or use a tampon for three weeks. Worst of all, her atypical Pap smears are never far from her mind. Could she have a serious condition? Why does she keep having atypical Pap smears if her biopsies look normal? Is she facing a lifetime of atypical Pap smears? Why isn't this a problem for any of her friends?

Jeannie's concerns are understandable. There are few situations more frustrating for patients, clinicians, and pathologists alike than repeated atypical Pap smears that remain unresolved. In the previous chapter, we briefly discussed the concept that atypical changes seen on a Pap smear are not specific for HPV. In fact, the majority of atypical Pap smears are onetime "random" events in a woman's life and appear to be caused by such diverse conditions as infections, pregnancy, and hormone use such as oral contraceptives. For many women with atypical Pap smears, it is never clear what caused her cervical cells to look atypical, but whatever the inciting cause, its effects are temporary. Other women, like Jeannie, are not so lucky.

If you have been in Jeannie's situation, you are undoubtedly all too familiar with the frustration of being repeatedly told that your Pap smear is atypical but a straightforward diagnosis cannot be made. To make matters worse, most clinicians (and pathologists) will not want to repeat an atypical Pap smear immediately in order to let the cervix "rest" and heal the minor trauma of the previous Pap smear procedure. Immediately after a Pap smear is taken, your cervix will show reactive changes that can obscure any changes due to HPV. For women so situated, this may mean months of uncertainty before their test is repeated. To paraphrase one of our patients with this history, this is "a real drag."

While the situation of repeated ASCUS Pap smears can happen to anyone, as pathologists we are aware that women in certain "groups" tend to have problems with atypical Pap smears. In this chapter, we will discuss some of the special circumstances that can lead to a woman having multiple atypical Pap smears that may have nothing to do with HPV infection. Although an atypical Pap smear *always needs further follow-up with your physician or clinic*, in some situations, a woman's Pap smear is less a reflection of her HPV status than it is her special life circumstance, as we will discuss later in this chapter. We will also discuss the situation when a woman is given a definitive diagnosis of a SIL but her biopsies do not show the lesion seen on her Pap smears. This situation is called a *discordant* or noncorrelating Pap smear and biopsy and can also lead to diagnostic uncertainty.

THE PREGNANT PATIENT

Most women will have a Pap smear taken at their first obstetrician's visit when their pregnancy is confirmed. As mentioned earlier, this Pap smear is rarely optimal since the practitioner will likely avoid the transformation zone in order not to disturb the endocervical canal. Remember, the transformation zone is the primary site of SILs resulting from HPV infection. But since the endocervical canal needs to stay tightly shut during a woman's pregnancy in order not to dislodge the fetus, this is generally a wise trade-off. Hence, many pregnant women will have a Pap smear that is "satisfactory but limited by lack of endocervical cells." This is considered acceptable in a pregnant patient.

Most women with a history of normal or BCC (benign cellular changes) Pap smears need not worry about a limited Pap smear when pregnant. However, if a woman has had a history of abnormal Pap smears, her clinician may elect to perform several Pap smears during the course of her pregnancy as extra insurance that she is not harboring a high-grade precursor or a cervical cancer during her pregnancy.

Another problem encountered with pregnant patients is their propensity for developing nonspecific atypical changes just by virtue of their being pregnant. Pregnant women can have Pap smears in which the nuclei in their cervical cells become larger, darker, and more irregular. The cause is thought to be the sea of high-octane hormones that wash through a woman's body when she is pregnant. These hormones contribute to the many annoying symptoms that pregnant women experience (and also to maintaining her pregnant state!) but they can also cause unseen changes in cervical squamous and glandular cells. Obviously, abnormal changes in a pregnant woman's Pap smear can also be due to HPV-related effects. However, compared to a nonpregnant woman, it can be relatively harder to prove or disprove the existence of HPV-related changes since her Pap smear "normally" can look quite atypical.

Remember from chapter 4 that repeated atypical readings generally lead to colposcopy (examination of the cervix with a lighted instrument) and biopsy, which involves taking a small bit of the cervix for tissue examination by a pathologist. Since colposcopy involves nothing more than inspection of the cervix, this can be performed safely in a pregnant woman. Because of the key importance of not disturbing the cervix during pregnancy, cervical biopsies are generally taken very judiciously. It is usually strictly avoided unless there is some suspicion from the cells on the Pap smear that either a high-grade SIL or cancer is present. An endocervical curettage is never performed during pregnancy.

In general, a pregnant woman with an atypical report will be treated very conservatively, especially if this is her first atypical report after a long history of negative Pap smears. For many women, their pregnancy-related atypical Pap smear results vanish after the birth of the child. When due to the hormonal fluxes of pregnancy, these results typically vanish without a trace and a postpartum Pap smear, usually taken six weeks after the delivery, is normal. In some women, it may take longer for their Pap smears to revert to normal.

IUD-RELATED EFFECTS

Another well-known cause for atypical Pap smears is the "IUD effect." An IUD or intrauterine device is a small metal or plastic contraceptive placed within the uterus to prevent pregnancy. The device has a string attached which comes out through the cervix to assist in its removal. The IUD in the uterus can lead to bizarre cells on a Pap smear by virtue of its effect on the endometrial glandular cells (the cells that line the uterus). The device may cause these cells to ball up and occasionally demonstrate atypical nuclear changes. These cells then "fall" into the vagina through the cervical opening and are picked up and smeared on a Pap smear slide. Endocervical cells may also show these atypical changes. Correct interpretation of these cells is helped by the clinician giving the laboratory information about the presence of an IUD when a woman has one in place.

Another problem seen in women with IUDs is that occasionally, the device will harbor a bacterial infection known as "actinomyces." On a Pap smear, these groups of bacteria resemble unruly balls of navy blue silk thread. These colonies of bacteria occasionally are spread over much of the slide making it difficult to see the underlying cervical cells. In this instance, a Pap smear will be deemed "limited for interpretation" with a comment about actinomyces. If present, some clinicians may elect to treat this infection.

The IUD string that comes through the cervix can also produce changes in cervical cells that may be seen on a Pap smear. The minor irritation of the string on the cervix may result in a finding of "parakeratosis." This is a benign change which in most instances reflects surface irritation. It can also be seen in an older woman whose uterus is dropping into the vagina (uterine prolapse) producing a chronic rubbing of the cervix. With a finding of parakeratosis, it is helpful to know its cause (IUD, prolapse, etc.). Parakeratosis may also be a finding in SILs and it is important to exclude that possibility.

HORMONES FOR CONTRACEPTION

The birth control pill is a more popular method for contraception than the IUD. It contains synthetic hormones that work by fooling the body into thinking it is pregnant. Given the occasional difficulty in interpreting a pregnant woman's Pap smear, you might expect that the oral contraceptive pill (OCP) may lead to the same type of difficulties. As in pregnant women, these potent female hormones can occasionally cause the cells of the cervix to have larger and darker nuclei. This situation is further complicated by studies showing that a woman's chances of developing a SIL seem to be increased when she is using birth control pills. Therefore, it is prudent not to ignore any atypical results in women on the pill. However, if you are on the pill and have been the recipient of multiple abnormal Pap smear reports, be aware that some women will consistently show atypical cells on their Pap smears. These atypical smears usually lead to colposcopy and biopsies. If the results of these studies are normal, the atypical results most likely represent the effect of the birth control pills.

There are other popular forms of hormonal contraceptives that are not taken as a pill. One example is Norplant, a slender rod containing hormones which is inserted under a woman's skin on her upper arm. In this site, it continuously releases pregnancy-preventing hormones into the blood for up to five years. Another example is Depo-provera, a hormone contraceptive injected into a woman every three months. These are very convenient forms of birth control in that there is no need to remember to take a daily pill. Both Norplant and Depo-provera are well known for producing characteristic changes on a Pap smear. Pap smears from young women on these forms of contraception will often look as if they were taken from a woman who is much older with atrophy or age-related changes. Sometimes mild atypical results can be seen on smears due to the hormonal effect and are not HPV-related. It is important that the clinician let the laboratory know when a patient is using one of these birth control methods. This is information that should be included on the Pap smear requisition form that accompanies a Pap smear from a doctor's office to the laboratory.

We have discussed the changes hormone contraceptives can produce on Pap smears, all of which might lead to an atypical result. However, bear in mind that while hormones may be responsible for atypical results in these settings, the largest group of women to use contraceptives (twenty- to thirty-year-olds) is also the age group with the highest incidence of SILs. The problem of contraceptive hormone effect on top of a precancer can be very difficult to sort out.

THE POSTMENOPAUSAL PATIENT

The woman who is perimenopausal (approaching menopause) to frankly menopausal (this can be roughly between forty and sixty years of age) will experience changes in her body that relate to the decline of sex hormones. There is an abundance of good information in the lay press and other sources on the many physical and emotional changes that accompany this period leading up to the menopause. What many women may not know, however, is that their Pap smears are likewise affected, mirroring what is happening to other parts of their bodies. As a woman experiences the sometimes startling effects of her diminishing sex hormones, the cells of her reproductive tract, including the cervix, are likewise undergoing unseen changes.

Most of these effects have to do with "atrophic" or "thinning" changes in the cells that line the vulva, vagina, and cervix. It is these changes that can lead to the uncomfortable feelings of vaginal dryness that many women experience during this period. On a microscopic level, the layers of squamous cells (epithelium) lining a woman's vulva, vagina, and cervix become thinner and the individual cells themselves also change. The cells become relatively smaller causing the nuclei within them to become relatively larger. Nuclei can also become darker. Recall that similar changes are also seen in cells infected by the HPV virus.

Since most pathologists who examine Pap smears are aware of these changes, atrophic smears are usually recognized as such and are called normal. However, in some postmenopausal women the changes become extreme and it is difficult to decide whether an HPV-related lesion is present or if we are looking at a case of "atrophy-related atypia." In some unusual instances, these changes can even mimic cancer. These age-related changes are particularly worrisome in this population of older women since if they actually did represent HPV-related changes, they may have persisted for many years, long enough to progress to cancer. As mentioned previously, most cervical cancers are seen in older women who have long-neglected HPV precancers.

Older women with this category of atypical Pap smears luckily have an option other than that of waiting for (sometimes multiple) repeat Pap smears. In many instances, a woman's postmenopausal atypical results can be made to go away by treating the woman with a short course of topical estrogen cream over a period of a month followed by a repeat Pap smear. This hormone cream inserted into the vagina will generally reverse the atrophy and cause the squamous cells in the cervix to "mature up," that is, look less like atrophied cells. If the atypical changes seen are due to hormonal effects, these changes should vanish with estrogen treatment. If the changes seen are due to an HPV-related lesion, these abnormalities will still be present on a repeat Pap smear. In exceptional circumstances, a woman's cells will not respond to hormonal therapy and it will still be unclear whether she is harboring HPV. In these instances, HPV testing may be helpful in determining whether a persistent HPV infection is present (see chapter 9).

Another problem encountered with postmenopausal women has to do with the common symptom of vaginal dryness which torments many women. You will remember from chapter 3 that failing to spray the cells on a slide immediately will result in "air-drying," which can lead to Pap smears erroneously interpreted as "atypical." In menopausal and postmenopausal women, air-drying is very common due to the peculiarities of atrophied cells. This compounds the problem of atypical reading due to atrophy because it is even more difficult to correctly interpret air-dried cells. Again, the application of estrogen cream over a month seems to do the trick of "reversing" both the cause of atrophy-related atypical results and the air-drying that usually accompanies it.

Many women decide to undergo hormone replacement therapy either to alleviate menopausal symptoms or to provide long-term protection against heart disease (although this is now controversial) or thinning bones. This therapy has the added benefit of relieving atrophy-related changes on the Pap smear. However, because of the many effects, good and bad, of taking hormones, women would do well to research the risks and benefits of hormone use in their own particular case and discuss this issue with their physicians.

Many women take "natural" hormones, such as the plant-derived preparations called "phytoestrogens," two plant sources being soybeans and ginseng. These may be sold in health-food stores or on the Internet. If so, it is a good idea to let your physician know this. She will want this information to assess any symptoms you may have, such as vaginal bleeding, as a result of these medications, and the laboratory also needs to be informed of each patient's hormonal status in order more accurately to interpret their Pap smears.

WOMEN WITH REPEATED ATYPICAL RESULTS

Whether you belong to any of the above-mentioned groups or not, you may end up having multiple or repeated atypical Pap smears like Jeannie. As we have seen, you can have a totally innocuous cause for your atypical Pap smear such as hormonal effects or inflammation; however, if the changes produced are pronounced enough, you may be facing many years of "atypical" readings on your Pap smears. Thankfully, this is a rare occurrence. Women in this category resign themselves to almost always receiving an atypical report and are prime candidates for HPV testing (see chapter 9).

Marcy, one woman we interviewed, said that her physician would call her to tell her that she had an atypical Pap smear, but she would let Marcy know if it was her "normal abnormal" Pap smear rather than an "abnormal abnormal" Pap smear. While she undergoes periodic colposcopies as well as biopsies, for the most part, she is used to getting an ASCUS reading on her Pap smear. No one is sure why this keeps happening, but fortunately both she and her clinician are comfortable handling this situation.

NONCORRELATING PAP SMEARS AND BIOPSIES

The situation of a "noncorrelating" or discorrelate Pap smear and biopsy is one in which you receive a diagnosis of SIL on your Pap smear but your biopsy is normal. This particular situation is potentially even more vexing than that of receiving repeated atypical Pap smears. In this case, although you have been given an unambiguous diagnosis of SIL on your Pap smear, no HPV-related lesions can be found with colposcopy and biopsies. Since you cannot go forward with treatment for a SIL without a tissue (biopsy) confirmation of your diagnosis (see chapter 4), this result leaves you and your clinician dangling. What could cause this situation?

One possibility is that your clinician did not biopsy the correct place on your cervix and you have a SIL that still needs attention. This can happen either because the lesion is very small and is not readily visible even with the magnifying aid of a colposcope. It may also occur because your SIL is obscured by other problems such as infection and it is difficult to determine the correct area to biopsy. Lesions high in the endocervical canal can also be difficult to detect. Women in this situation may need a repeat colposcopy and biopsies or even a loop excision (see chapter 4). Occasionally a SIL diagnosed by a Pap smear is never found by biopsy or loop excision. We can only speculate that the SIL regressed (disappeared) in the time between the Pap smear and biopsy. This is particularly probable in cases of LSIL since roughly 60 percent of LSILs go away on their own in one to two years.

Then again, your Pap smear may be "overread" by the laboratory. In other words, changes on your Pap smear that may be interpreted as "atypical" or even a SIL to one laboratory may be interpreted as "reactive" or "atrophic" (and hence benign) to another laboratory. This may reflect the experience of the laboratory handling your Pap smears. Also, we have previously mentioned how very subjective a Pap smear reading is. In chapter 8 we give you some guidelines for discussing with your clinician the particulars of the laboratory chosen to read the tests.

If you are a woman with repeated and unsolvable atypical results or non-correlating Pap smear and biopsy reports, you can ask your clinician to have the laboratory "re-look" at your atypical Pap smears, especially if the subsequent cervical biopsy is normal. In view of your normal biopsy, perhaps they can be reinterpreted as favoring a reactive diagnosis. Some laboratories do this automatically and give the clinician a "correlative statement" on their reports. This statement attempts to correlate or interpret both the Pap smears and biopsies together. This is very powerful and can help make sense of puzzling discrepancies, particularly if they are persistant.

Occasionally, it may make sense to request a second opinion, especially if you have had multiple atypical Pap smear reports and one or more sets of negative biopsies. Ask your clinician for a recommendation of a second laboratory for another opinion. Look for a laboratory involved in diagnosing a large number of Pap smears and biopsies every year. It is helpful if the pathologist reviewing your case is Specialty Certified in Cytology, a subspecialty of pathology. This is usually the case at large laboratories or academic (university) centers. Finally, women with discrepant or puzzling Pap smear and biopsy reports are another group who may benefit from testing for the HPV virus. The pros and cons of HPV testing will be addressed in chapter 9.

Up to this point, we have discussed the role of the Pap smear in detecting cervical SILs and thus preventing cervical cancer. Unfortunately, not all cervical cancers are caught in the precancer stage. Rarely we are called to make a diagnosis of cervical cancer. In the next chapter, we discuss cervical cancer, what the diagnosis means, its treatment, and the outcome of this disease.

S I X

Cervical Cancer

DEALING WITH THE DIAGNOSIS

U ntil now we have been advising you about your abnormal Pap smears and biopsy results with the hope that any changes that may have taken place in your cervix are benign or at least have remained in the *pre*cancerous stages of cervical dysplasia or SIL. However, what do you do if you are a woman who has been given a diagnosis of cervical cancer? Even though much progress has been made in cancer diagnosis and treatment, for many people, the word "cancer" evokes a series of frightening images that inevitably end in death. Even the idea that you may have to deal with a malignancy is a difficult one to accept.

While neither of your authors has ever had cervical cancer, we have had the misfortune of dealing with cancer diagnoses in immediate family members. Between our two families, we have experienced surgical removal of a tumor, radiation therapy, cancer chemotherapy, and the entire spectrum of roller-coaster emotions that serious illness brings to bear. But both of us have also had the extreme good fortune of having our family members survive and pass the "five-year cancer-free mark." From our personal experiences and from our professional lives as pathologists, we are here to tell you that individuals can survive their cancer diagnoses and go on to lead long full lives. In this chapter, we will walk you through the stages of dealing with cervical cancer, from the initial shock of receiving your diagnosis to discussions of further treatment options to suggestions for getting through the crisis. While cervical cancer is the "worst-case scenario" of an abnormal Pap smear, when detected at an early stage, it is also one of the most successfully treatable cancers.

115

RECEIVING A CANCER DIAGNOSIS

The women we have spoken to with cervical cancer have been unanimous in stating that the shock of receiving a cancer diagnosis was almost the worst part of their ordeal. Even though most women are aware that their Pap smear is being taken in order to check for cancer, it still comes as a shock to hear the "C word."

Jennifer, a thirty-year-old newlywed, is still in disbelief over her cervical cancer diagnosis. She had an abnormal Pap smear five years ago but in her pursuit of a busy career that involved a lot of traveling, she neglected to follow up that Pap smear result. Some nonspecific gynecologic complaints led her to make an appointment to have a routine exam. At that exam, she was shocked to hear her doctor say that her cervix looked suspicious for cancer. He recommended her to an oncologist, a cancer specialist. Jennifer was unaware that she was at-risk for cancer and thought that she was too young for the diagnosis. She left her exam with many questions milling around in her head. Was she going to die? Could she still have children one day? Was she going to need surgery or chemotherapy?

Deborah, a fifty-three-year-old grandmother diagnosed with cervical cancer, had never had a Pap smear in her life. She was told that she wouldn't live out the year. Would she really not live to see her grandchildren grow up? What was in store for her?

According to the American Cancer Society, in the year 2000, an estimated 12,800 women in the United States received a diagnosis of invasive cervical cancer. Each year, roughly 5,000 women die from their disease. Statistics from the National Cancer Institute indicate that both the incidence (number of cases) and mortality (death rate) from cervical cancer have declined about 40 percent since the early 1970s. In the early '70s, about 75 to 80 percent of serious cervical diagnoses were for invasive cancer with the remainder being "preinvasive" (SILs).

Today, thanks to early detection of cervical precancers by the Pap smear, that ratio is reversed and only 20 percent of serious cervical diagnoses are for an invasive cancer. In fact, the majority of women with cervical cancer today are women who have either never had a Pap smear or haven't had one in the past five years. Most of these women are over forty years old and have had long-neglected HPV-related precancers.

You will recall that the hallmark of cancers is their ability to invade and destroy normal tissue. Later they may also gain the ability to move throughout the body via the bloodstream or lymph vessels. Just a brief comment on terminology: some pathologists and gynecologists use the term "carcinoma-in-situ" to describe a kind of high-grade SIL. Even though the word "carcinoma" appears in the diagnosis, this is not the same as invasive cancer or invasive carcinoma. "In-situ" refers to the abnormal cells remaining confined to their usual location on the surface of the cervix. They have not as yet gained the ability to break through the tissue boundaries that normally contain them, a tight collection of collagen strands known as the "basement membrane." It is only when the basement membrane is breached by the abnormal cells that the process of "precancer" becomes an invasive cancer and a diagnosis of malignancy can be made.

For most of the discussions in this chapter we will be talking about squamous cell cancer, which is the most common type of cervical cancer. We will discuss adenocarcinoma, a cancer of glandular or endocervical cells, as well as other more unusual types of cancers later on in this chapter.

What are the symptoms of cervical cancer? Very often, the woman is symptom-free as is generally the case in women with precancerous lesions. However, cervical cancer can produce symptoms, most commonly vaginal bleeding at unusual times, such as between periods or after intercourse. A woman with cervical cancer can also develop a vaginal discharge, which can be pink-tinged or frankly bloody or she can even experience massive vaginal hemorrhaging.

In the absence of symptoms, a diagnosis of cancer might be suspected from visual examination of the cervix on a routine exam. Because a cancer can break through the surface covering of the cervix, the cervix can appear eroded or ulcerated and will be "friable," which means that it bleeds easily, sometimes spontaneously, with intercourse, or at the mere touch of the physician's instruments. Occasionally, the tumor will appear as an obvious mass that protrudes out into the vagina. Rarely, the cancer will not be obvious on the surface of the cervix but will have extensively involved the "body" of the cervix so that it feels enlarged and abnormally firm (sometimes called "barrel-shaped"). A physician who encounters areas that appear suspicious for cancer should perform biopsies of these areas regardless of the Pap smear result. These biopsies will then be sent to the laboratory where a cancer diagnosis can be made.

Occasionally, the tumor will not be obvious on a simple pelvic examination. This may be because the mass is hidden up in the endocervical canal or because the cervix is inflamed or contains benign polyps that are small non-cancerous growths. In some cases, an invasive tumor is small and can only be identified by looking into a microscope at a biopsy specimen. When a cervical cancer is not obvious to the examining physician, a Pap smear may be the first indication of a malignancy.

Some cancers are easy to diagnose as malignant on a Pap smear. These cases will be read as either "suspicious" or "positive" for malignancy by virtue of the characteristic features of the cells. Often, however, the Pap smear will be read as an HSIL since a cervical cancer can shed cells that appear identical to those seen with high-grade SILS. In these cases, since a diagnosis of HSIL on a Pap smear leads to a colposcopic examination, the actual diagnosis of a cancer will be made with a tissue biopsy taken during the colposcopy (see chapter 4). The colposcope greatly magnifies features of the surface of the cervix so that subtle changes in the surface or the presence of atypical-appearing blood vessels can alert a gynecologist to a cancer. These suspicious areas can then be biopsied.

Occasionally, a cervical cancer will produce a diagnosis of "atypical cells of undetermined significance" (ASCUS). This is because the tissue debris and blood characteristic of cancers can obscure the malignant cells sufficiently so that they cannot be definitively diagnosed as malignant although they are still recognized as atypical. In most instances, these cases will be diagnosed as "ASCUS, favor a HSIL," or otherwise indicate a worrisome atypical result, which should trigger the same follow-up colposcopy. Biopsies taken at the colposcopic exam would then confirm the cancer diagnosis.

It is no exaggeration to say that receiving a cancer diagnosis is a shock. You should be receiving the news from your gynecologist in person. He or she will then likely refer you to a specialist unless your usual gynecologist also happens to specialize in gynecologic cancers. Your gynecologist will likely attempt to answer some of your questions about the diagnosis and try to give you some idea of what to expect. Unless your physician is very well versed in recent therapies of cervical cancer, however, he or she may not be able to give you a detailed accounting of what to expect next. Much will depend on your specific diagnosis as determined from your pathology report. Also of great importance are the results of any clinical "staging." These are tests performed to determine if your tumor is confined to the cervix or has spread beyond it. Examples of cervical cancer staging are given later in this chapter.

In any case, for most patients, this first visit is primarily for absorbing the initial diagnosis rather than for much decision making or even information gathering. As one patient with cancer said to us, "After my doctor said 'cancer,' I couldn't hear the rest of his explanations, nothing else he said that afternoon made much sense." Another patient told us, "I had to eventually stop him from talking. I told him that I could hear words being spoken and I could see his lips moving but I couldn't understand what he was saying." At the end of this chapter, we will be giving you some suggestions to help you navigate through this trying time in your life. In the next few sections, we will be providing you with some factual information.

HOW CERVICAL CANCER SPREADS

Cervical cancer generally spreads by invading nearby tissues in the area of the cervix where it first arose. The tumor may first invade the adjacent vagina and uterus and then later, if unchecked, spread to tissues outside the uterus such as the bladder and rectum, which is the end portion of your colon. Advanced cervical cancers are notorious for blocking the ureters, the tubes that connect your kidneys to your bladder which can cause urine to back up into the kidney and later damage it. Cervical cancer can also cause your bowels to be obstructed due to compression by the tumor. While these effects on nearby organs are serious, the gravest problems occur when cervical cancers invade blood and lymph vessels. This allows the cancer to spread more widely, to lymph nodes in the pelvis as well as to distant organs such as the lungs and liver.

CANCER STAGING

A crucial element in deciding your therapeutic options as well as your prognosis (chance of recovery) is the "stage" of your cancer. The staging system most commonly used in this country is based on a system devised by FIGO, the International Federation of Gynecology and Obstetrics. A summary of this staging follows. You will note that some of the stages are further subdivided into "A" and "B" forms.

Stage 0: Carcinoma-in-situ or HSIL (precancer)

Stage I: Invasive cancer that involves the cervix only

Stage IA: A small amount of cancer is present which is not seen with the naked eye but only by using a microscope

Stage IB: A larger amount of cancer as seen using a microscope or by using the naked eye and which is confined to the cervix

Stage IB1: Cancers no greater than 4 cm in size

Stage IB2: Cancers greater than 4 cm in size

Stage II: Cancer has spread beyond the cervix but is still inside the pelvic area

Stage IIA: Cancer has spread to the upper two-thirds of the vagina

Stage IIB: Cancer has spread to the tissues surrounding the cervix (parametrium)

Stage III: Cancer has spread throughout the pelvic area. The tumor involves the lower third of the vagina or the tumor has caused a blockage of urine from a kidney to the bladder (ureteral obstruction)

Stage IV: Cancer has spread to other parts of the body

Stage IVA: Cancer has spread to the bladder or rectum (nearby organs)

Stage IVB: Cancer has spread to distant organs such as the lungs

CERVICAL CANCER STAGING: HOW IS IT DONE?

The information regarding the extent of spread of your tumor will come from many different types of tests, some will be familiar to you from past instances of medical testing and some will be new. It is critical that the physicians involved in your care try to get as accurate a picture as possible of how much of your body is involved by tumor since this information will guide therapy in your individual case. The following is a list of some of the types of staging procedures that your physicians may want you to undergo. Not everyone will require all these tests. If your tumor is very small and superficial, for example, you may not be required to have any testing beyond the original surgery you had to make the diagnosis.

Blood Chemistries: These tests are the familiar blood tests that you are likely to have had many times before. Of particular interest to your doctor are the BUN/creatinine tests that look at kidney function. These tests may be altered if the tumor compresses the urinary tract. Liver-function tests are also performed since these may be elevated if the tumor has involved the liver. Calcium levels may also be elevated if a patient's bones are involved in advanced-stage disease.

Chest X ray: An X ray is done to determine if there are any tumor masses in the lungs (metastatic disease) from the cervical tumor. Although it is extremely unlikely in early-stage disease and not very common even with late-stage disease, lung metastases would radically alter your course of therapy.

Examination under anesthesia (EUA): This is a pelvic and rectal examination done while you are asleep under a general anesthetic. This allows the examiner to do a more thorough examination of the lateral (side) portions of the vagina and the tissues surrounding the cervix. This study is often done during surgery so that you will not have to undergo anesthesia separately for this procedure.

Intravenous pyelogram (IVP): This test looks at kidney function and is performed by injecting a contrast agent into the bloodstream that then becomes concentrated in the kidneys. An X ray taken after a period of time will show the agent in the kidneys and indicate either normal or abnormal kidney function. This is important since all cases with abnormal kidney function (unless it can be shown to be due to other causes) will be assigned to Stage III even if according to other clinical findings, the patient appears to be a Stage I or II. The abnormal kidney function in these cases is assumed to be due to the tumor involving and blocking one of the ureters, the tube leading from the kidney to the bladder.

Computed tomography (CT) scans: These studies use computer-assisted X rays with a high resolution to visualize the internal organs, particularly the lymph nodes, which are difficult to see any other way except with surgery. Lymph nodes may be enlarged if they contain metastatic tumor. CT scans can be useful in determining the extent of tissue involvement beyond the cervix in higher-stage cancers. A CT scan with intravenous dye can also be used to look at kidney function and is often used instead of an IVP to assess kidney function.

Cystoscopy and Sigmoidoscopy: These two studies are performed in women to confirm more advanced or higher-stage disease or in planning radiation therapy. Cystoscopy involves using a lighted tube to visually inspect the inner lining of the bladder for tumor involvement. Likewise, sigmoidoscopy examines the inner lining of the rectum and lower colon to check for tumor. If either the bladder or rectum are involved the tumor stage will be assigned as Stage IVA.

CANCER TREATMENT: THE PHYSICIAN SPECIALISTS

You may have three different physicians treating you during your cervical cancer therapy, reflecting the three kinds of treatments available for the disease. "Oncology" is the general specialty of treating cancers. An oncologic surgeon is the physician, typically a gynecologist with specialized training in cancer therapy, who is responsible for removing the cancer in an operation. This is usually the first line of therapy you will be receiving. Some cancers will benefit from radiation therapy (using high-energy rays to kill tumor cells) administered by physicians called "radiation oncologists." Medical oncologists are the physicians who administer cancer (drug) chemotherapy.

TREATMENT OPTIONS FOR CERVICAL CANCER

Generally, cervical cancer is treated either by removing the uterus and cervix with pelvic lymph nodes (these are collections of immune cells and also the first stop for metastatic cancer cells) or by radiation therapy. Under some circumstances, radiation therapy or chemotherapy is given first before surgery. Two factors determine whether you will end up having surgery only or surgery with some combination of chemotherapy and/or radiation therapy. The first is your clinical stage. The lower or less advanced the stage of your cancer, the less likely it has spread and the less therapy is usually needed. The second factor is the customary treatment for your stage of cancer in your region of the country. Like many other facets of medicine, therapies for cancer can vary quite a bit depending on where you live and whether or not you have access to a regional cancer center.

Surgical Treatment

Surgical treatment of cervical cancer has been around since the 1800s. The procedure used most often today is the radical hysterectomy. This operation is performed through an incision in the abdomen. The uterus, cervix, upper portion of the vagina, and the tissues around the cervix are removed along with the pelvic lymph nodes that primarily "drain" the cervix and may harbor metastatic cancer cells. To avoid the necessity of having to take replacement estrogen hormones, in younger, premenopausal women, the ovaries can be left in place. Older women will usually have their ovaries removed. The mortality rate from the surgery is low (less than 1 percent with experienced surgeons).

Complications of this surgery mostly center around difficulty emptying the bladder after surgery. The bladder lies on top of the uterus and must be dissected away, thus various nerves leading to the bladder can be damaged. Less commonly, difficulty having bowel movements occurs as a result of nerve damage. Other complications are the same as for any other type of major surgery and include blood clots to the lungs and problems with bleeding or infections after surgery.

Recuperation time varies with each woman and will depend on factors such as age, the general state of physical health prior to surgery, and if any complications occurred either in surgery or afterward. Usually, to protect the bladder, a catheter is left in place for at least a week and your doctors and nurses may teach you how to empty your bladder using a catheter. This guarantees that the bladder is never too full until the affected nerves heal. Similarly, stool softeners (like Metamucil), a high-fiber diet, and an increased intake of water can help in preventing severe constipation. Suffice it to say that this is a major trauma to your body and you should expect to take a while (weeks to months) to fully recover and feel like yourself.

Some women express concerns about the loss of sexual function, such as problems with orgasm, occurring after cervical cancer therapy. This is particularly of concern with hysterectomy. A woman's perception of herself as a sexual being is critical for good sexual function after treatment. As one gynecologic oncologist told us, "Orgasms are more related to what is in your head than what is between your legs!" Also of critical importance is the attitude a woman's partner has toward her cancer and her body. Some men are fearful of hurting a woman "down there" after treatment for cervical cancer. If your partner has an aversion to sex after therapy, chances are you will not be enjoying it much either.

Some women may have problems with pain during intercourse because of a narrowing of the vaginal canal (vaginal stenosis). Other women may have issues with decreased estrogen production if their ovaries are removed in the course of surgery. This could result in a "surgical menopause." These are problems that your doctor can help with, either through estrogen replacement, vaginal dilators, or other medications.

Radiation Therapy

The goal of radiation therapy is to deliver a high dose of radiation to the cervix and vagina in order to destroy the cancer cells while minimizing the dose received by the bladder and rectum. These two organs suffer the most complications with this type of therapy. Generally this is most often done by using a combination of "external" beam radiation and "internal" or transvaginal radiation.

External beam whole pelvic radiation is usually performed during a four- to five-week span of time. With this type of therapy, radiation is directed to your pelvis from the outside. You will be lying on a special table after first having had tiny "tattoo" marks placed on your skin so the beam of high-energy rays is always directed to the same spots. You will be having the treatments at an outpatient facility and can come and go between therapy sessions. Generally, women receive their radiation treatments five days a week with weekends off.

Another method of getting a high dose of radiation to the cervix while sparing the other pelvic organs is the transvaginal or intracavitary radiation. To accomplish this, a transvaginal applicator is generally placed in the patient while she is under general anesthesia. The applicator consists of a tube placed in the uterus through the endocervical canal along with two oval or cylindrical devices that fit against the top of the vagina. The applicators are then loaded with radioactive sources.

With this type of therapy, a woman is usually hospitalized and isolated in a special lead-lined room for one to three days during which she needs to remain immobile. Women we have spoken with report that this can be the toughest part of their therapy. The isolation and immobilization are difficult for many women to bear. Some of the newer radioactive sources are more powerful and permit shorter exposure times. With these powerful sources women need not be hospitalized for transvaginal radiation therapy.

Complications of radiation therapy are due to the effects of radiation on normal tissues, typically the intestines and bladder. Both acute (immediate) and chronic (late) reactions can be seen. Acute reactions typically include diarrhea and nausea.

Late complications occur in 5 to 15 percent of patients and include inflammation (cystitis) of the bladder, which can cause the need to urinate frequently; painful urination; or blood in the urine. These symptoms are caused by radiation-induced scarring of the bladder and can be seen a year or more after therapy. Treatments exist for this condition but it can be a difficult ordeal and involve washing the bladder with special solutions and medications. Late effects of radiation on the bowel can also occur after a year or more and can include diarrhea, constipation, or bleeding from the rectum.

Another late complication sometimes seen is shortening or narrowing of the vagina (vaginal stenosis). This may be alleviated by sexual intercourse or frequent pelvic examinations to break up the thin fibrous scarring that can develop. This condition can also be helped by using a molded plastic dilator to stretch vaginal tissue.

Another potential complication of radiation therapy involves a woman's ovaries. Efforts will be made to shield the ovaries from the effects of radiation for the purpose of preserving their hormone function. If a premenopausal woman's ovaries are irradiated, they will shut down within a week of the start of treatment at which time she would begin to experience menopausal symptoms. This would be a permanent change which, depending on her age, may necessitate sex hormone-replacement therapy. Whether their ovaries are shielded or not, women who receive pelvic irradiation for cervical cancer are not able to later become pregnant. Even the smallest doses of radiation will destroy the reproductive ability of the ovaries.

One additional potential long-term complication of pelvic irradiation for cervical cancer is that of secondary malignancies. These are malignancies that women may rarely experience solely as a side effect of radiation. This is because radiation can act to cause tumors as well as cure them. Because these organs are in the area that receives radiation, a woman's bladder, rectum, and ovaries are at approximately twice the risk for tumors compared with women who have not received pelvic irradiation.

Cancer Chemotherapy

An important change in the treatment of patients with cervical cancer is the use of chemotherapy at the same time as radiation therapy. Chemotherapy, which decreases the bulk of the tumor, may be given prior to surgery but in most cases is given along with radiation therapy. Chemotherapy may shrink the tumor so that it is easier to remove surgically or to irradiate. An added benefit is that chemotherapy may kill cancer cells that have spread beyond the pelvis. These cells are usually not targeted with radiation and would escape its effects.

The most commonly used chemotherapeutic agents in cervical cancer are platinum-based compounds such as cisplatin. The most commonly seen side effects are nausea and vomiting. Less common side effects are ringing in the ears, some selective hearing loss, and kidney damage. It is rare to lose your hair with this drug.

THERAPY BY CANCER STAGE

Stage IA: At this earliest stage of cervical cancer, the tumor invades to a depth of less than 5 mm as measured on the glass slide under the microscope. Generally, a diagnosis of cervical cancer at this early stage is unsuspected and it is usually made on a cone-biopsy specimen (see chapter 4) performed because a woman was thought to have had a high-grade SIL. On the cone-biopsy specimen, there is usually an extensive HSIL, but at a few points, the cells have just started to invade the underlying normal tissue by breaking through the basement membrane. This type of cancer is known as "minimally invasive" or "microinvasive" cervical cancer.

If the depth of invasion is less than or equal to 3 mm as measured on the glass slide, recent studies indicate that the cone biopsy is likely to be adequate treatment if the "margins" of the cone biopsy (the surgical "edges") are free of HSIL or cancer. At this level of invasion, the likelihood of metastatic disease is 1 percent or less. This is the only tumor stage where the treatment (cone biopsy) will still allow a woman to keep her uterus and conserve her fertility. It is absolutely critical in these patients that a regular Pap smear schedule is religiously maintained, however. It may even be prudent to have scheduled colposcopies to ensure that there are no recurrences. Obviously, a hysterectomy can also be done, especially if the woman is done with child-bearing.

Stage IB and IIA: In patients with Stage IB tumors (confined to the cervix, larger than Stage IA tumors), either surgery or radiation may be used. In general, patients who have the best results with surgery are patients whose tumors are small (Stage IB1) and who are healthy enough to undergo the stresses of surgery. Patients with larger tumors (Stage IB2) who undergo hysterectomy have a higher risk of having metastatic cancer cells within their lymph nodes and are likely to require radiation after surgery. Many oncologists feel that the evidence strongly points to chemoradiation (chemotherapy *and* radiation at the same time) as the therapy of choice for any locally advanced cervical cancer beginning with Stage IB2 tumors (see treatment for Stage IIB and Stage III tumors, below).

For patients with Stage IIA tumors (involving the upper two-thirds of the vagina, without involvement of tissue outside of the cervix), therapy usually depends on the extent of vaginal involvement. Patients with tumor extending deep into the vaginal tissues are usually not considered to be good surgical candidates. Again, although there are regional variations in cancer therapy, chemoradiation is becoming the treatment of choice.

Stage IIB and Stage III: Patients with extensive disease are not generally considered to be surgical candidates. Since it is difficult to completely remove the tumor surgically without also having to remove other vital organs, options for these patients in some parts of the country include radiation therapy or chemotherapy prior to radiation. In early 1999, the National Cancer Institute released a report of five large studies that seem to indicate that better results may be obtained with chemoradiation. This is becoming standard therapy in some parts of the country. Although it is not clear what the best drugs are, they likely will be platinum-based. Some patients may undergo surgery after chemoradiation if residual tumor is present.

Stage IVA: Patients with cancers of this stage have tumor involvement of their bladder or rectum. Treatment options include extensive surgery known as a "pelvic exenteration" which removes the pelvic organs (uterus, bladder, lower bowel) in one large block. Since a pelvic exenteration removes the bladder and lower bowel, this results in a woman requiring both a colostomy (stool empties into a bag on the abdomen) and a nephrostomy (urine also empties into a bag on the abdomen). High-dose radiation therapy is also an option and allows the pelvic organs to be preserved. Chemoradiation again is becoming the standard of care in some parts of the country.

Stage IVB: These patients have cancer at distant sites (metastatic disease) and will need to have chemotherapy since their disease, at this stage, involves areas away from the pelvis. These patients can also receive radiation therapy to relieve pain or other symptoms of their cancer.

CANCER SUBTYPES

Generally, when we are talking about cervical cancer, we are speaking about the most common type of cancer, squamous cell cancer (or carcinoma). This is because the most common type of precursor lesion is the SIL or squamous intraepithelial lesion, which, as we are well aware, arises from squamous cells in the cervix. However, as we have mentioned, cancers can also arise from the endocervical or glandular cells of the cervix. This type of cancer is called "adenocarcinoma." This type of cervical cancer will be discussed in more detail in the next section of this chapter.

Other types of tumors, although rare, can also occur in the cervix. "Lymphoma," a tumor of a type of white blood cell, can originate in the cervix, as can "melanoma," a malignancy that we usually associate with skin lesions. A particularly aggressive form of cervical cancer is small cell (or small cell undifferentiated) carcinoma. This is a type of cancer that is usually seen in the lungs of smokers but can appear in other organs as well. Another unusual type of cervical tumor is the "sarcoma," which is a tumor not of the lining cells of the cervix, but of the underlying "support" cells.

Women with unusual cervical cancers are generally at a disadvantage since there is not as much clinical data supporting the use of one treatment over another since there are so few women with these tumors. If you have been diagnosed with an unusual subtype of malignancy, it is important that you be treated at a specialized cancer center since they will likely have more experience with your type of tumor.

ADENOCARCINOMA OF THE CERVIX

As we have discussed earlier, the human papillomavirus infection that leads to cervical cancer can also target endocervical cells. The precursor lesion is adenocarcinoma-in-situ (AIS), which was discussed in chapters 3 and 4. The invasive counterpart of AIS is invasive adenocarcinoma. This tumor type accounts for 10 to 20 percent of all the invasive cancers of the cervix. This cancer can be difficult to detect since it arises in the endocervical canal and tends to spread both upward toward the uterus as well as "inward" to involve the body of the cervix. It is thought that this tumor may be less sensitive to radiation than squamous cell cancers so some clinicians advocate a combined approach using both radiation and surgery.

CERVICAL CANCER AND DES PATIENTS

Diethylstilbestrol (DES) was a hormone drug taken by pregnant women in the 1950s as a treatment for threatened miscarriages. Women whose mothers took DES when pregnant with them (DES daughters) have a small (less than one-tenth of 1 percent) but real risk of developing an unusual variant of adenocarcinoma called "clear-cell" cancer in their cervixes or vaginas. These women need to be particularly vigilant about their Pap smears and inform their physicians about their DES exposure. It is currently unclear, however, whether they are at increased risk for run-of-the-mill SILs and squamous cell cancers.

CERVICAL CANCER AND PREGNANCY

Discovering a cervical cancer during pregnancy can transform a joyful time into one filled with anxieties. Although a pregnancy will not hasten the course of cervical cancer or worsen the prognosis, if a woman chooses to wait until the baby is born before beginning her therapy, it will delay treatment. In the case of an early (before the third trimester) pregnancy, a woman can choose to abort the fetus and continue with cancer therapy. When the diagnosis is made later in pregnancy, typically the infant is delivered by Caesarean section or vaginally when the fetus is able to live on its own. If a Caesarean section is performed, a hysterectomy can be performed at the same time if considered necessary and a woman does not want more children. For more extensive cancers, radiation therapy may be necessary instead of, or in addition to, hysterectomy.

RECURRENT CERVICAL CANCER

There are probably few experiences as disheartening as finding out that your cancer has come back. Of those that recur, the vast majority (80 percent) do so in the first two years following initial therapy. After five years, recurrences can occur but they are rare. As you might expect, recurrence rates increase with higher-stage cancers. While only 10 percent of Stage I tumors recur, up to 70 percent of Stage IV will return after initial therapy. The treatment for a recurrence will depend on the type of treatment previously given and the extent and location of the recurrent disease.

EXPERIMENTAL APPROACHES TO CERVICAL CANCER

In addition to the standard therapies available to women with cervical cancer, experimental treatment protocols are also available. These options are generally offered to women with advanced disease who have perhaps failed standard therapy. The protocols usually originate from different agencies such as the National Cancer Institute and the Gynecologic Oncology Group. More information about these protocols can be garnered from their respective Web sites (see Appendix B).

The therapeutic vaccines (discussed in chapter 11) are an example of an experimental therapy. Other options include experimental chemotherapy drugs, the use of different types of drugs called "biological modifiers," as well as other novel molecular compounds. In order to qualify for a particular protocol, women usually need to fulfill strict "eligibility requirements." These pertain to tumor stage, prior therapies, age, and type of tumor among other characteristics. Occasionally, however, if a woman is not responding to conventional therapies and will clearly die without some sort of therapeutic intervention, she will be given experimental therapy for "compassionate use" even if she does not fulfill protocol requirements.

ALTERNATIVE APPROACHES TO CERVICAL CANCER

What about alternative therapy for cervical cancer? At the current time, nothing outside of conventional cancer therapy has been convincing for reducing cancer mortality. Is there anything wrong with using herbs or massage or Chinese medicine for treating cervical cancer? If a therapy is not dangerous in that it does not require you to forego any recommended therapy from your doctor and it makes you feel better about your condition, then it is likely doing you more good than harm. It is wise to clue your physician into whatever additional medicines or herbs you may be taking. Bear in mind that, occasionally, even "harmless" botanical or herbal remedies have negative interactions with conventional medicines.

The only real danger lies in using unproven therapies to the exclusion of therapies which have been shown to work. This can result in dangerous delays in beginning your cancer therapy. Unfortunately, there are a lot of hucksters who prey on frightened individuals by offering miracle cancer therapies. It doesn't take a genius to figure out that any miracle remedy out there would have been patented and released by some multinational drug company by now! The proliferation of chat rooms and message boards devoted to alternative therapies has made it that much harder to separate the wheat from the chaff. We recommend sticking to the conventional therapies for cervical cancer for now. The stakes are too high.

Although somewhat controversial, there are some dietary supplements that should be taken with caution during treatment for cancer. You may want to ask your oncologist about vitamin C, in particular, since some researchers believe it may actually benefit some cancers. This was reported in 1999 by scientists at Memorial Sloan-Kettering Cancer Center in New York who looked at the effects of vitamin C on cancer cells. Antioxidant vitamins in general, such as vitamins C, A, and E should be taken cautiously during radiation therapy. Antioxidants act by destroying "free-radicals" (compounds produced in our bodies which are discussed further in chapter 10). Radiation therapy, however, does its job by creating free radicals that act to destroy the cancer being irradiated. There is concern that ingesting these vitamins could reduce the effectiveness of radiation therapy.

CERVICAL CANCER: GETTING THROUGH THE CRISIS

Receiving a diagnosis of a serious illness like cervical cancer is, to put it mildly, a major life crisis. While cancer cells are assaulting your body, emotions like grief, fear, anger, and disbelief are assaulting your mind. However, unlike other crises you may have navigated in the past, a medical crisis involves grappling with unfamiliar terminology and uncomfortable and deeply invasive procedures all taking place in the sterile and decidedly unsoothing environs of a hospital. As survivors of numerous crises, medical and otherwise, we offer you the following seven strategies for managing a cervical cancer diagnosis.

1. Educate yourself

Learn about your diagnosis. Read what you can about the disease and ask questions of all the professionals with whom you come in contact (although don't get carried away, see strategy 5, below). Often, you'll find that nurses and physicians' assistants have more time to address your concerns. Your physician will undoubtedly have pamphlets and fact sheets on the specific aspects of the therapy you will be undergoing or can recommend good sources of literature. Take notes during your appointments and ask questions later. One patient we spoke with, an educator, recommended that a good way to end a visit with a physician is to ask, "Are there any questions that I haven't asked but should have?" Or, "Are there any questions that the typical patient asks that I haven't yet asked?" Appendix A provides a list of questions that you may want to ask about your cervical cancer.

Other good sources of information include the American Cancer Society, which can often provide names of cervical cancer patients whom you can contact for firsthand information. The Internet is also teeming with good resources although, because Web sites are not regulated, you need to be careful and check the source of any information you come across. (Don't forget, the Internet was responsible for widely distributing the "helpful health advice" that bras cause breast cancer!) We list informational Web sites that we found to be helpful in Appendix B at the end of this book.

2. Acknowledge that you are in the midst of a crisis and ask for help as needed

If you are like most women in the twenty-first century, particularly if you are holding down a job and have a husband with some kids and a pet or two for good measure, your own well-being is likely to be at the very bottom of your to-do list. Probably somewhere after "pick up the laundry" and "take the dog to the vet." To garner the resources to handle a serious illness like cervical cancer, you will need to quickly move yourself up to the top of that list. That's right. For once, it is going to have to be about you! You need to train to get better as though you were training for an athletic event. You will need to eat as nutritiously as possible and get sufficient rest. Whenever possible, you should get as much stress-reducing exercise as you can. In fact, some physicians suggest that this may hasten your recovery from any procedures you might undergo. Many women find solace in spiritual pursuits during trying times, whether they are more traditional like going to church or more introspective like writing in a journal or practicing yoga. There are even meditation tapes available for cancer patients to guide them through healing imagery. This is a practice where women can visualize their cancer being attacked by their immune cells, chemotherapy drugs, or radiation. Women can further visualize their tumor shrinking and even disappearing with hopes that it will actually do so.

It is vital that you ask for what you need, whether it is help with the children or some time with a close friend or a hug from your partner. This is not the time to be shy or self-sacrificing. Your survival may depend on you asking for what you require of others, and your happiness with or without cancer absolutely requires it. Also, look to "nontraditional" sources of support. One woman with cervical cancer derived great comfort from her radiation therapy technologist who consistently told her that she would be fine.

As important as it is to seek out the positive aspects of your life, it is critical to avoid the negative energy drains that we all have. Treat negative people like the plague. You do not have the luxury of shouldering the problems of the sad sacks of the world and wondering endlessly about other peoples' agendas. More important things must concern you. Be selfish. Your life may depend on it.

3. Find a buddy

One patient we spoke with who has been through the trial of repeated atypical Pap smears and multiple colposcopies (although thankfully not cervical cancer) recommends bringing a buddy with you to your appointments. She states that someone like a close friend or sister may even be better that a husband or significant other because they may not be as emotionally invested as a partner might be. We think this is excellent advice. It is very difficult to listen and formulate questions while trying to remain calm and emotionally in control at the same time! It is probably safe to say that no more than half, if that, of information given in a doctor's office can be heard and digested, particularly if that information is of an upsetting nature. Having a second set of ears can be a useful reality check later for answering questions like "Did she really say . . . ?" or "What did she mean by . . . ?" Not to mention the comforting effect of having someone there to support you or even to help you find your car in the hospital parking lot! The right advocate can make your endless round of appointments much easier to bear. Give your friends the privilege of showing you how much they care.

4. Don't be afraid to seek a second opinion

Getting a second opinion is a pretty commonplace event in medicine these days and in the case of cancer therapy, it is usually covered by most health insurance companies. In particular, you should consider seeking another physician's opinion if your cancer is at an advanced stage, particularly if it is metastatic. If you are about to embark on experimental cancer therapy, you might want to seek someone else's opinion. Also, if you are a cervical cancer patient in a "special" category such as someone who is pregnant or perhaps with an unusual type of tumor, it may be a good idea to seek a second opinion. Ideally, you will be getting your second opinion from a specialist with a reasonable amount of experience and who sees a lot of patients in your situation.

5. Choose the "right" doctor

Choosing the right doctor very much depends on the individual since one woman's decisive doctor is another woman's arrogant jerk! Remember that this is the person with whom you will be sharing both good and bad news. This is also someone with whom you may be discussing some very private concerns such as your sexuality after treatment. Obviously, you will want someone competent but we think two great qualities in a doctor are great listening skills and kindness. Certainly, you should feel comfortable asking questions and expressing your concerns. You should never be made to feel uncomfortable asking for clarifications at any point. Remember, the only dumb question is the one not asked.

Once you have decided on your doctor, we would advise guarding against second-guessing his or her suggestions. While you should absolutely feel free to express your concerns, ultimately, you are going to have to trust this person to help you become healthy. We know it is difficult for some of us to give up control but it is exhausting to try and manage your own illness. You will be doing yourself a disservice if you become your own doctor. While you will want to be as well-informed as possible, don't attempt to read all the primary medical literature on the subject. There is just too much material and it is too confusing to analyze and compare complicated medical studies. Unless you are a professional medical epidemiologist, you will need someone to interpret the data for you. It is your physician's job to condense the information and present it to you so that together you can make the best possible treatment choices.

6. Make use of your hospital's and community's resources

Many resources are out there for cancer patients although it might take a little searching to find what is right for you. Your hospital is probably the best place to start. Generally, a hospital that is taking care of a sizable number of patients with cancer will be able to provide you with resources such as support groups and perhaps regularly scheduled lectures on topics pertaining to therapy. The American Cancer Society also has support groups in various cities across the country. Lastly, the Internet is a source for support groups, some of which are specifically targeted to women with cervical cancer. We include these resources in our Appendix B.

7. Cultivate a positive attitude

Several women we talked to with advanced cervical cancer stressed the importance of positive thinking in their battles against cancer. One woman was able to clearly visualize becoming well for her family. This woman, while squarely facing the possibility of her own death, decided that it would not be her fate. While this may not totally explain her long-term survival, it surely did not hurt.

DEATH FROM CERVICAL CANCER

Despite everyone's best efforts, the woman's as well as her physicians', some cervical cancers are either too far advanced or too aggressive to be treated successfully by the therapies discussed above. The overall death rate from cervical cancer is highly stage-dependent. Stage I cervical cancers have a remarkable survival rate of 90 percent after five years but only 30 percent of women with Stage IV tumors survive five years after their initial diagnosis.

Women who are terminally ill with cervical cancer usually experience the effects of their tumor on vital organs. Kidney function can fail and total obstruction of the bowel may occur. Massive liver involvement with tumor can cause coma and death. Some women succumb to complications of their therapy.

Women who are dying of their disease need to be surrounded by people who care about them and can help them through their final days. Supportive family and adequate nursing help are critical. Every effort should be made to allow a woman to die in her own home rather than in a hospital. Cancer centers usually have personnel trained in hospice care, the special care of terminally ill people. These centers can provide hospice referrals to ease the difficulty of a woman's last days.

By now you have received a wealth of information about Pap smears, SILs, and cervical cancer. In the next chapter we provide a glimpse into the lives of several women who shared how they were affected by their cervical disease. Hopefully these accounts will provide insight, support, and encouragement for your experiences with your abnormal Pap smear.

S E V E N

Women's Stories

W e were inspired to write this book as a result of numerous conversations with women about their abnormal Pap smears and cervical abnormalities. We were astounded at the deep and often lasting effects that these issues had on their lives. Many of these conversations occurred casually as friends, colleagues, and sometimes strangers approached us to ask about some aspect of their diagnoses or to seek reassurance about a given Pap smear report. Several of these women agreed to grant us more extensive interviews.

We also enlisted the aid of some of our clinical colleagues who introduced us to patients who have undergone the various procedures that we have written about in this book as well as women who were diagnosed with cervical cancer. We are grateful to all these women, many of whom gave generously of their time to speak to us. They honestly told us of their fears for their health, their relationships, and their sexuality. Many of them wanted their stories included in this book in the hope that other women would not have to endure some of the difficulties that they did. We are indebted to these women and offer a sampling of some of their stories in this chapter although we have incorporated other women's experiences throughout this book. We have changed names and life circumstances to protect their privacy.

CANDY, A TWENTY-YEAR-OLD WAITRESS WITH HSIL

Candy first learned of her abnormal Pap smear last year when she saw a gynecologist in order to get a prescription for birth control pills. She got his name from a friend who had also just started seeing him. After that visit, she received a phone call at home from her physician who told her that she would need to come in for colposcopy and biopsies. She was told that she had moderate dysplasia (HSIL). According to Candy, she did not understand what this meant and her doctor could not explain the term to her in a way that made sense. Although she knew that she would have to come in for a second appointment, she was not sure why.

At her appointment, Candy tried to discuss her diagnosis with her physician but again did not completely understand his explanations. She was told that she had contracted the HPV virus sexually, which was something like the herpes virus. She felt that he was communicating that this "was all a bad thing, a sexually transmitted disease." She felt that her physician saw her as promiscuous. Although the colposcopy and biopsies were not painful, she left the procedure in tears feeling deeply ashamed.

Although Candy is close to her mother, it was a while before she could summon the courage to tell her mother about her diagnosis. Candy felt that she had a shameful secret. Her physician gave her some pamphlets in his office but these were all "in medical terms." According to Candy, "The pamphlets used big words to explain other big words and it all meant nothing to me." It was still not clear to Candy what she had and how it was related to a sexually transmitted disease.

Fortunately, Candy's mother happened to have a friend who was a cytotechnologist and could explain the significance of HPV and cervical dysplasia. Candy also was grateful that her mother's friend appeared pretty matter-of-fact about her diagnosis and gave her some sense of the large number of women who were in the same situation she was with abnormal Pap smears and a diagnosis of SIL.

After Candy received her diagnosis of dysplasia on her biopsies, she went in for another doctor's appointment. At this appointment, she was better informed thanks to explanations provided by her mother's friend. She was able to actively discuss the next step with her physician. He recommended a hospital loop procedure in about a month.

Candy had the procedure under general anesthesia and spent the rest of the day sleeping. She took a total of four days off to recover. Once the procedure was over, Candy breathed a sigh of relief; she felt sure that her problems with her cervix were over. However, at her first postloop Pap smear, she again learned that she had an abnormal Pap smear. This time, instead of calling, her physician sent her a card that said to schedule an appointment to discuss a Pap smear abnormality. On the bottom of the card, he had written, "Use condoms when having sex." Candy was at the time living with her boyfriend and she did not understand what her physician meant. Did he mean that she could pass HPV to her partner? Did he think that she was having sex with other men and would pass it on to them? And why would he communicate such sensitive material in such an impersonal way?

Candy was also under the impression that once you "took out the bad part, it was gone." She didn't realize that her dysplasia could return or that she could still have abnormal Pap smears.

After receiving what she felt was an insulting card from her physician, Candy decided that she would not return to that gynecologist. She went to her primary-care doctor for a repeat Pap smear. This one came back as normal. At the appointment with her primary-care doctor, she wanted to have an IUD inserted. Her doctor, however, could not get the device up through her cervix and suggested that she might have some scarring in her cervix due to her loop procedure.

Candy wants to know if she will ever go back to a normal life. Is she now more at-risk for abnormal Pap smears? Will her cervical scarring cause future problems with conceiving a baby? Will she have problems with the pregnancy if she does get pregnant?

What is clear from talking to Candy is that the lack of a well-developed relationship with her physician made the news of her cervical abnormalities much harder to bear. Unlike some of the women with whom we spoke, Candy had very few difficulties with pain associated with her procedures but she suffered deeply nonetheless. Because of her belief that HPV infections were rare, she at first felt embarrassed about discussing her ordeal with anyone, including friends and family. She is now left wondering if she will be dealing with complications for a lifetime because of an infection that she didn't even know she had.

What kinds of advice might we give Candy? First of all, it is essential that she find another gynecologist to continue her necessary Pap smear follow-up. Because of her bad experience with her first gynecologist, she will want to carefully choose her new doctor and ask friends and relatives for recommendations. She may want to consider scheduling a visit or interview of sorts to any potential new doctor to see how her many concerns are addressed. Once she decides on a new physician, Candy may want to bring along a friend or relative for support during their initial appointment.

MELISSA, A WOMAN IN HER LATE TWENTIES WITH HSIL

Melissa is a strikingly pretty young woman with a soft, throaty voice. She is bright and articulate but like most of the young women with whom we spoke, she had not heard about HPV or its relationship to cervical precancers when she first developed her abnormal Pap smears. Because her mother had had some sort of gynecologic problem that led to an early hysterectomy, Melissa thought that her cervical problems might be genetic. At one point when she wondered about the cause of her problems, her gynecologist responded by saying, "We're not going to worry about the cause, we're worrying about the solution." When we asked if she was able to get her questions answered by her clinicians, she stated, "I really didn't even know what to ask." It was only after she had done some research on her own that she came to realize that she had been exposed to HPV.

Melissa received her first abnormal Pap smear report while she was still a college student. She remembers that they were alternately normal and abnormal, "flip-flopping" back and forth for about half a year. At that point, she was told to have a Pap smear every month. After five months of abnormal Pap smears, they finally became normal and she was able to move to a regular schedule of Pap smears. Everything was quiet until her senior year of college when she once again had an abnormal Pap smear.

She then had a cervical biopsy and was told that she had an "abnormal growth" on her cervix which proved to be an HSIL that needed to be removed. Two weeks later Melissa had laser surgery. This went well and she felt great afterward, even going back to work the next day. Six months later, a checkup revealed that her lesion was back, as large as when she first had it removed. At this point, she was scheduled for "old-fashioned scalpel surgery." Although she was in and out of the hospital in one morning, she felt the procedure for days. She described it as being very painful and the whole experience really made her wonder what was going on with her body. She then was put on, as she describes it, the "high-maintenance" doctor schedule. This required her to see a doctor for a Pap smear every three months for two years and then every six months for the next two years before going to a yearly schedule. She has had normal Pap smears since then.

Melissa is an example of a woman who sought out information herself after not being offered any as a patient. She wonders if something about her body made her susceptible to the effects of the virus and has been seeking the advice of a naturopathic physician who is an alternative healthcare provider. Although Melissa has taken charge in an admirable way, there are still many unanswered questions for her. She wonders if her HPV infection is putting future children at-risk for disease. She wonders if she is exposing future sexual partners to HPV. And most importantly, is she now free of HPV?

Unfortunately, Melissa is a fairly typical example of a young woman who is told very little about the cause of her cervical disease, even after she directly asked for an explanation. Once she discovered the sexual origin of her condition, she understandably became concerned about the future ramifications of her diagnosis and what it meant for her as a sexual partner and a future mother. We can reassure Melissa that with so many negative Pap smears since her treatment for HSIL, it is highly likely that her body has gotten rid of her HPV infection. Of course this is not to say that she could not become infected by a different HPV subtype from a new partner. As for the issue of future children, this should not be a problem for her unless her cone biopsy procedure has induced cervical scarring or cervical incompetence. While investigating alternative practices such as naturopathy may be helpful, we do strongly recommend that Melissa remains religious about having an annual Pap smear.

MARCY, A LAWYER IN HER MID-THIRTIES WITH REPEATED ATYPICAL RESULTS AFTER TREATMENT FOR HSIL

Marcy is an outspoken woman with an easy laugh and a straightforward manner. She was aware when in high school that she needed close gynecologic follow-up since her mother told her that she was a DES daughter. At about the age of twenty, she had her first abnormal Pap smear, which was a "mild dysplasia" (LSIL). At that point she had an in-office cryotherapy procedure to freeze the abnormal areas off her cervix. She let her visits to a gynecologist lapse while she was in college and it was only after her sister insisted that she begin regular checkups that she saw a gynecologist once again.

At this next checkup, years after her cryotherapy, she was dismayed to once again have an abnormal Pap smear. Her cervical disease by now had progressed to a moderate to severe dysplasia (HSIL). At this point, she required an in-hospital cone biopsy. Marcy was able to enlist the aid of family members to come and see her through the procedure. She then started receiving follow-up Pap smears every three months at first and then every six months. These were all normal until two years after her cone biopsy when she once again began receiving abnormal Pap smear reports.

In marked contrast to Melissa and Candy, Marcy was lucky to have a physician who communicated closely with her. Marcy always got a handwritten note from her doctor along with her abnormal Pap smear diagnosis to indicate how concerned her doctor was with any given Pap smear report. Since Marcy very often had abnormal Pap smears, her physician would let her know whether her Pap smear was a "normal abnormal" report (that is, normal for her) or an "abnormal abnormal" report. These notes were very helpful for Marcy. According to Marcy, because she and her physician *had established a relationship*, she trusted her doctor to use her judgment to decide what needed to happen next. Importantly, Marcy always felt that she understood this decision-making process.

Marcy pretty much continued to have Pap smears every three to six months. Many times she would need to make a second appointment for colposcopy depending on the degree of abnormality of her Pap smear report. At some of these colposcopic exams, she would have biopsies taken, all of which were normal. On one visit, she had a loop excision of her cervix.

After a while, all of the procedures on her cervix made Marcy nervous about future fertility since she had heard that repeated cervical procedures may make getting pregnant and retaining that pregnancy difficult. Since she was at a point in her marriage where she was thinking seriously about having children, Marcy decided to get pregnant. Fortunately this happened without difficulty. An unexpected side effect was that her Pap smears were all normal during the course of her pregnancy. She did not get away from close medical follow-up, however, and ended up having thirty-four office visits during thirty-six weeks of pregnancy! Marcy jokes that she might have been better off getting an apartment next to her doctor's office.

Despite what sounds like an ideal relationship with her physician, the repeated visits to her doctor's office impacted Marcy's life. Fortunately, Marcy's law practice was flexible enough that she was able to schedule her medical appointments with relative ease although she acknowledged that this would likely present problems for women who did not enjoy as much flexibility in their jobs. All in all, Marcy has had an appointment with her gynecologist every three to six months for eight years.

Recently, her physician has used the HPV test to check for the presence of HPV in her cervix. Marcy recalls that this test was negative, which has allowed her physician to cut back on her return visits.

For Marcy, the most significant issues have been scheduling repeated doctor's visits into her life as well as "the worry before and after." Much of her ordeal has been made bearable by having an excellent rapport with her doctor and getting personal feedback from her instead of an impersonal call from the office. Several times during our interview, Marcy emphasized that she could *rely on her physician's judgment*. This offered her a degree of comfort that her doctor was doing all that Marcy needed as well as keeping Marcy informed of what the next steps would be.

As far as dealing with the worry, Marcy stated that she tried not to think too much about the diagnoses but would deal with whatever came up as it unfolded. She was also fortunate in having a very supportive family. Marcy was adamant about the need to have a support person, either a family member or a girlfriend, whenever "something new" came up such as the need for colposcopy or an ultrasound during pregnancy.

Because of Marcy's long-term relationship with her physician and her many years' experience with cervical procedures, she has helped her physician in "teaching sessions" with medical students and nurses who are trying to learn cervical colposcopies and biopsies. This "educational" aspect also makes Marcy feel better since she is contributing to the education of health professionals by her example as a patient. Marcy also emphasized the need for more widespread dialogue about HPV and cervical dysplasia since the more women know about these issues, the more they will know what to ask their healthcare providers should they receive the news that they have a cervical abnormality. Marcy is an example of a patient who has taken charge of her own health care by being informed and asking for support from her family and others. She is also extremely lucky to have a physician with whom she enjoys a close and supportive relationship.

Marcy is also an example of a patient who has taken charge of her cervical issues despite the inconvenience of multiple medical visits and the chronic "worry" surrounding those visits. Marcy illustrates our belief that there is nothing like a supportive relationship with your clinician to ease the stress of repeatedly abnormal test results.

JODIE, A YOUNG WOMAN WHO
WAS MISDIAGNOSED WITH CANCER

Jodie is an educated young woman with a calm demeanor. She felt guilty for many years because she neglected to have a Pap smear. She thinks that she had equated having Pap smears with being sexually active and since she had not dated anyone for awhile, she thought it was not necessary to have a Pap smear. When she finally did go in for a test, she was surprised to get a call from the office informing her that it looked "irregular." She had no idea what that meant. But after calling several friends who all said that they had had an abnormal Pap smear at one time which turned out to be nothing, she felt reassured.

Jody was referred to a gynecologist, but when she arrived at his office she was shocked to find out that he planned to take biopsies of her cervix. She had no idea why she was there and no one had told her that tissue would be taken. The biopsies "hurt like bloody hell" but what was even worse, when the doctor took a look at her cervix, he let out a breath and said, "Oh, boy!" This comment stayed in Jodie's mind as she waited for the biopsy results to come back.

Jodie called several friends including one who was a cancer survivor, who helped to calm her down. Her friend was able to explain the process of obtaining biopsy results from the lab. Four days after her procedure, Jodie was called into the doctor's office. Jodie described her physician as appearing extremely nervous. His mouth trembling, he began by saying, "Well, I guess you know why you're here." Jodie said she told him that she had no idea why she was there. At that point, her doctor told her she had "adenocarcinoma, a rare and serious form of cervical cancer." He also told her to cancel everything in the foreseeable future and that she would probably never have children. She left shaken, in tears. The rest of the day was a blur. Jodie remembers spending most of it on the telephone with friends. She called work and said that she had no idea when she would be returning.

Jodie had an appointment with an oncologist at a cancer center two days later. She arrived in an anxious state, but had brought a friend with her. In contrast to the gynecologist who had given her the initial diagnosis, the oncologist had a comforting and soothing demeanor. He immediately calmed her down by acknowledging her nervousness and told her, "Your cancer doesn't scare me. It's not the usual type that we treat but that doesn't mean that I'm any more scared by it." She felt her fear slowly subsiding as she took in his words. He also described her probable treatment options, which might just consist of a cone biopsy, and not a hysterectomy. This news was a huge relief.

Jodie went home and prepared to have surgery in a few weeks. She was so overwhelmed by her diagnosis that she could not even go online to read up on her cancer although she asked some friends to do so for her and "filter" the information. Because her tumor was thought to be small, she ended up having a cone biopsy.

Her cone biopsy shocked her with the amount of pain she felt once she came out of general anesthesia. She spent nine hours in the recovery area with a friend while the nurses helped her with pain medications. She stayed at home for a week after the surgery.

After her operation, Jodie was given the great news that her original biopsy slides had been misdiagnosed as adenocarcinoma and the cone biopsy actually showed an adenocarcinoma-in-situ, a noninvasive precancer. However, this lesion was at the margins (edges) of the cone biopsy, which meant that she required a second cone biopsy. Before this second procedure, she spoke with friends and did some research on pain associated with these biopsies to see if there was some way to deal with the intense pain she had previously experienced. She requested that her physician give her a local anesthetic in addition to a general anesthetic which she said made her second cone biopsy much less painful.

All of this has happened in just the last year. Jodie feels, in some strange way, that her experience was a useful life lesson. It has taught her not to react to every little thing that happens in life because she now knows that things could change in an instant. Having survived a roller-coaster ride that took her from malignancy to precancer and then back to health, she has learned not to "ride the waves" but to maintain an even balance. Her suggestion for someone in a similar situation is not to panic over every new development but to take a slow breath and try to approach the situation with calmness and balance. This is probably a good outlook for whatever we face in life.

When Jodie spoke with us, she was in the midst of "shopping" for a new gynecologist. After her ordeal with her first gynecologist, she wants this person to be calm, kind, and informative. Since her initial experience, Jodie is now very well educated in cervical matters and knows what questions to ask should she ever encounter another abnormal Pap smear. Jodie's experience also demonstrated the importance of speaking with as many people as possible whenever she was scheduled for a new procedure. The aggregate experience of her wide network of friends helped her deal with each new twist and turn as it surfaced.

DEBORAH, A LONG-TERM SURVIVOR OF ADVANCED CERVICAL CANCER

Deborah was fifty-three years old when she was diagnosed with cervical cancer. She credits her strong sense of independence and pride in helping her survive this devastating disease. The mother of ten children, she says, "I had never had a Pap smear in my life." In fact, Deborah's first Pap smear was performed when she saw her doctor for worsening vaginal bleeding. She had been bleeding lightly but continuously for a number of months but the day she experienced massive vaginal bleeding, she knew something was wrong. Her doctor looked at her cervix, took her first Pap smear and a cervical biopsy, and told her that he was concerned she may have cancer.

That was the start of Deborah's long battle with cervical cancer. Deborah told us of her cancer story seated in her living room. One wall of this room is completely covered with photographs of all of her children, her sixteen grandchildren, her parents, and other loved ones. She frequently digresses from her cancer story to talk of her children. It is clear that her family is a very strong presence in her life and was an important factor in her recovery.

When she returned to see her doctor later that week for her test result, her worst fears were confirmed. Deborah's physician handed her the test results and then left her alone to read her results while he ran an errand. The report was filled with large words she didn't understand. A nurse came in to see how she was doing and Deborah asked the nurse to help her read her report. "Is it cancer?" Deborah asked. The nurse told her it was and the two of them read the report together making sense of all the new medical terms.

The results told Deborah she had invasive squamous cell carcinoma of her cervix. When her doctor returned from his errand, he asked the nurse how she took it. Deborah's doctor then told her she had about six to nine months to live. He told her he couldn't help her but would send her to the nearby university cancer center where she could be treated.

Deborah says she had been so worried about the possibility of cancer that the results didn't surprise her. Consistent with her matter-of-fact manner of dealing with life's adversities, she didn't seem unsettled that her physician presented her results in such an unusual manner. She went home and told her father the news that she only had months to live. He looked up from his gardening and told her she wasn't going to die, that "after all she had been through raising ten children, a little cancer wasn't going to kill her." Eleven years later, it looks like Deborah's father was right.

After receiving her cancer diagnosis, Deborah had an appointment at the university cancer center with a new doctor, a specialist in women's cancers. It was this doctor who sat down with Deborah and went over in detail what therapy she had in front of her and what her chances really were for beating her cancer. Deborah's cancer was fairly advanced so she was started on radiation therapy right away. She recalls the daily radiation therapy as being exhausting. She also recalls receiving some sort of chemotherapy at that time. Her tumor shrank and things were looking good. It was now a matter of waiting and watching to see if all of her cancer had been destroyed by the radiation.

Unfortunately, two years later, Deborah's cancer was back. Her doctor told her it was about the size of an orange and had spread to other tissues in her pelvic region. Now she would need surgery. Deborah underwent major surgery, one that removed just about all her organs in the vicinity of her cervix. Her surgery was called a "pelvic exenteration" and it took out her uterus, cervix, and ovaries, her bladder, and part of her colon including her anus. She now has a colostomy where she now passes stool into a plastic bag on her abdomen. Losing her bladder means that she doesn't urinate between her legs anymore but also into a bag on her abdomen, known as a "nephrostomy."

Deborah was in the hospital almost two months recovering from her surgery. Her children visited her every day while she slowly became stronger and learned to adapt to her new life. When asked about living with her changed body, Deborah responds strongly that she "has no time for self-pity." She doesn't dwell on sickness and she expresses impatience for others who do. It is clear that her strong will, refusal to feel sorry for herself, and her close-knit family had a lot to do with her life now as an active attractive woman with still a lot of living to do.

Eleven years after her diagnosis, Deborah's cancer has not returned and she can count herself cured of cervical cancer. She has minor ups and downs with her colostomy and nephrostomy, the latter being somewhat prone to infections. She prides herself on taking only one pill a day, that for her diabetes, and none at all that relate to her cervical cancer. That is behind her now.

When asked about her cervical cancer, Deborah knows now that Pap smears are a way to detect the disease early. Interestingly, Deborah volunteers that "none of my six daughters get Pap smears." She says she tells them that "they don't want to end up like me" but they don't get Pap smears because of their personal aversion to pelvic exams. She says she has never heard about human papillomavirus or the sexually transmitted nature of cervical cancer. This really isn't surprising given the time of Deborah's diagnosis in the late 1980s. The connection between HPV and cervical cancer wasn't confirmed until right around that time and later.

Deborah's story illustrates the absolutely critical importance of obtaining regular Pap smears. Her first Pap smear at age fifty-three was the one that told her she had cervical cancer. Despite this, her daughters still refuse to have Pap smears themselves. Deborah has had extensive surgery, radiation, and chemotherapy and has done well. Her strong family support, stubborn attitude, and refusal to indulge in self-pity have all contributed to her being a cancer survivor.

MARGARET, A NATIVE AMERICAN WOMAN WITH CERVICAL CANCER

From first learning of her diagnosis of cervical cancer, Margaret, a fifty-two-year-old Native American woman, knew she needed to draw deeply on her inner strength and spirituality as part of her battle against her disease. Margaret was alone, hundreds of miles from home at an Indian Health Service clinic, when she received the bad news. Margaret had never had regular Pap smears and it was well over five years since her last one. Margaret had the test at the insistence of her doctor. She had been having fairly continuous bleeding over the past few years which seemed similar to that experienced by other women friends her age. Her doctor had been trying to get her in for a

Pap smear for months but she always seemed to be bleeding, not a great time for a Pap smear her doctor told her. After almost a year, her doctor told her to come in for the test whether she was bleeding or not. She really needed to have a Pap smear.

Just looking at her cervix with her naked eyes, Margaret's doctor saw a very abnormal-looking cervix and told Margaret she was very concerned about the possibility of cancer. Her doctor took a cervical biopsy at that time and their fears were confirmed a few days later when the results of her biopsy were back. Margaret learned she had an invasive squamous cell carcinoma of her cervix. Her doctor immediately called the university cancer center, several hundred miles away, and told Margaret she had an appointment to be seen there the next day and that treatment would begin immediately.

Margaret was alone, without family members, when she received this devastating news. She was exhausted, unsteady with frayed emotions, and had a long drive ahead of her to her brother's home in northern New Mexico. Margaret sat alone in her car before she started the engine and tried to draw some strength from deep within. She thought of her family who needed her and composed herself for the long, lonely drive.

The next day Margaret told her family the news. One female relative, who Margaret describes as "very spiritually connected," prayed over Margaret. Margaret felt renewed by the prayers, "spiritually confirmed," and felt the strength to do "whatever it would take to get this cancer out of my body" using whatever her new doctor would suggest. Following her Native American traditions, Margaret began her daily "prayer of healing" which would sustain her through her ordeal.

The next day Margaret began six long weeks of combination radiation and chemotherapy. She took an immediate leave of absence from work, packed a few things from her home, and temporarily moved several hundred miles away for her treatments at the university. Her stepsister lived in this town and so at least Margaret had some family nearby and a place to stay.

Every day, five days a week, Margaret had radiation treatments. Once a week she had chemotherapy infusions. She recalls the experience as being "psychologically very traumatic, the most severe treatment ever imposed on anyone's body." She felt herself become increasingly weak and by her final weeks the chemotherapy was causing her nausea.

The clinics where Margaret received her care were very crowded and hectic with cancer patients, many with far-advanced disease. Her doctors were very caring but harried with little time for one-on-one support. She recalls speaking once to a social worker but it was the radiation therapy technician she saw daily to administer her treatments who supported Margaret through this time of "psychological torture." He assured her again and again that she'd come through it all, that she'd be okay.

The crowded and hectic cancer clinic was a difficult place to say and feel her healing prayer. Margaret found the need to extend her prayer to include all those working at the cancer clinic, her overburdened doctors, the harried technicians, and the support staff. Margaret says she "offered them all up with spiritual strength and guidance so they could help all of us," so they could be strong to help all of the patients recover. She included all the other cancer patients in her prayers. Margaret credits her Native American heritage for her strong cultural and spiritual beliefs. She felt "at the mercy of doctors but also God who has control over our lives." It was through her prayers she was able to feel involved in her cure and take some control over what she was experiencing.

Twice during the six weeks Margaret had radioactive implants inserted into her vagina to directly treat her cancer. For these treatments she was hospitalized in an isolated room with radioactivity-proof shields around her. For twenty-four hours each time she had to remain immobile on her back while the implant destroyed her cancer. She recalls that these periods were the most difficult for her of all her therapy. To sustain herself through this, she focused on her beloved grandson, less than a year old, for whom she wanted to live so that she could see him grow up and flourish. "I wanted to be there for my grandson, no matter what it took."

Margaret grew much closer to her family during this period. She and her stepsister had not seen much of each other in recent years but renewed their relationship during her therapy. She is thankful that her experience allowed her to reconnect with people in her life.

Now, over a year later, Margaret feels her life has changed forever. She feels good physically, although sometimes a bit tired. She has been back to work for almost a year. She says she eats much better now, focusing on fruits, vegetables, and grains, and drinks lots of water. She regularly meets with a local cancer support group that has become "my family."

The major impact on Margaret's life, however, is her renewed spirituality where she feels "keen awareness of everything around me." She says she "can't take anything for granted anymore." She feels life is "too connected and precious to ignore certain things" and she tries to make sure she "devotes attention to everything around me, from sunup to sundown." Margaret's grandson occupies much of her time when she is home. The two of them can't let a day go by without taking their walks, running, and playing. She remembers when she considered this time with him as a duty but now it is a tremendous pleasure.

Margaret feels renewed in all aspects of her life and actually feels grateful for the cancer having brought her to this spiritual place. She feels she "has been given another chance, another opportunity to live." She is also thankful for the sophisticated science and technology that was used to treat her.

After she finished her therapy and returned home to resume her life, Margaret had the unexpected shock of learning that the Indian Health Service would not be paying the medical bills for her cancer treatment. Such bills are typically astronomical and Margaret's were no exception. Through an unforeseen technicality, she was no longer eligible for coverage. Margaret has come to view this as just another part of her trials with cancer. She is determined to pay the bills herself, through her own earnings and by organizing fund-raisers at her current home and with her tribe. Once it is paid off, she would like to dedicate herself to further fund-raising for other unfortunate cancer patients who cannot afford their lifesaving treatments. She sees helping other people survive the ordeal she has survived as her future calling in life.

Margaret's story provides an excellent example of the value of family support, cancer support groups, religious beliefs, and personal inner strength in the fight against cancer. At the difficult time of her treatment, Margaret had the strength to turn her mental energies toward those helping her fight her disease. As a survivor, she tells us how cancer has changed her life for the better. Many other cancer survivors also relate how gaining a "second chance" at life allows them an invaluable and enriched perspective on their present and future life. Not surprisingly, Margaret is now devoting her energy to help others fight cancer.

CONSTANCE, A WOMAN IN HER FORTIES WITH RECURRENT CERVICAL CANCER

Constance is a forty-three-year-old female diagnosed with cervical cancer more than a year ago. She is an attractive, muscular, and very strong-appearing woman who looks the picture of health. During her adult life Constance inconsistently sought medical care and thinks it was over fifteen years since her last Pap smear. Her tumor was first detected when she experienced massive vaginal bleeding. "I thought I was going to bleed to death!" she recalls, and went directly to the local emergency room. When examined there, Constance's cervix appeared grossly abnormal and cancerous. One of the doctors told her she would die in three to five years. She remembers being furious with the physician. "How dare he say such a thing? How did he know? He wasn't God!" Even at this devastating moment she felt determined to fight the disease and live.

Constance associates her cancer with a gonorrhea infection she had twelve years ago. She thinks the tumor may have gotten its start around that time. On her own she has informed herself about cervical cancer and HPV and understands that other sexually transmitted diseases are risk factors for cervical cancer.

Constance had a cervical biopsy and its results confirmed the impression of invasive squamous cell carcinoma. She was referred to a university cancer center where she came under the care of an expert in female cancers. It was this doctor with whom she developed a close rapport and with whom she came to trust with her life. Constance agreed to the aggressive therapy her doctor outlined. She finally felt she had an ally in her fight.

A single woman with no children, except for her dedicated oncologist, Constance felt alone in her ordeal, so called upon her friends for support. She lived an hour away from the cancer center and knew she would need help getting to and from her treatment appointments. She "spread it around her friends," asking first one then another for help so that she didn't appear to be a burden to any one person. She was fortunate to have her sister come and stay with her for several weeks during part of her therapy.

Constance is a firm believer in nutrition, diet, exercise, and meditation as sources of strength and good health. With the approval of her doctor she embarked upon an "anticancer diet" with herbs, vegetable juices, brown rice, and green algae. She feels this diet helped her maintain her strength during her arduous treatments and that it helped her fight the cancer.

A radical hysterectomy was the first step in Constance's treatment. Her uterus, cervix, ovaries, and surrounding tissues were removed as were a number of lymph nodes. The pathology report from the surgery showed the tumor to be at a very advanced stage. It had extended well beyond the confines of the uterus and into the surrounding soft tissue. Most disturbing was the presence of tumor in numerous lymph vessels, even ones far from the cervix. As might be expected, Constance had numerous lymph nodes in the pelvic area with metastatic tumor.

Constance experienced extreme pain and weakness from the surgery. "I never thought it would hurt so much!" Her first few days after the surgery were the worst. It just didn't seem as though the pain medication was adequate. Once she recovered a bit, Constance began a combination of radiation and chemotherapy, receiving what she calls "the maximum of both." She had thirty sessions of radiation spread out over six weeks. Constance remembers how the radiation would leave a warm sensation in her lower abdomen. This was augmented with chemotherapy treatments given once a week.

Constance felt strong for the first few weeks but by the end of her combined therapy she felt "physically and emotionally devastated." The presence of her friends was critical for both physical and emotional well-being. Constance's animal friends were also a source of comfort, especially her dog. She recalls being so weak that she "barely had the strength to feed her chickens!" She recalls not being able "to do anything, not read, not eat, not anything." She lost weight and with a laugh says she "finally got rid of those pounds" she had been fighting for awhile.

It took four months after the completion of therapy for Constance to regain her strength and resume a normal life. She reports that once her strength came back, she has been full of energy, and now feels "totally fit." She is even helping build a house, an activity that requires a lot of physical strength on her part. She has continued her anticancer diet and has added antioxidants such as vitamin C and A to her daily regimen.

Constance had been finished with her treatments for a little over a year when recently she noticed a lump on her neck near her collarbone. It was an enlarged lymph node. She was due for a three-month checkup at the cancer center so at her appointment she showed her doctor the lump. The lump concerned her doctor. A quick biopsy was scheduled. The pathology results showed a lymph node with metastatic squamous cell carcinoma, this time at a site quite distant from her original tumor.

Both Constance and her doctor were understandably distraught over this bad news. "We have worked so hard to fight this cancer!" her doctor exclaimed. For it to return so soon in a distant site from her cervix indicates an aggressive tumor and one possibly difficult to treat. Constance underwent additional tests examining her lungs and bones to determine if there is more metastatic cancer than just the one lump. The examination showed a small nodule in her lungs thought to be another area of metastatic cancer.

After recovering somewhat from the shock of being told that her cancer had returned, Constance admits that her original cancer was so bad that she half expected this recurrence. Her doctor has started her immediately on an experimental protocol with further chemotherapy which will be more intensive than what she had previously. She is focusing her mental energy on "making the tumor go away" and says her enlarged node feels a bit smaller. She states with strong conviction that she will fight harder than ever for a cure. "I will not die from this," she states. "Look at me, I am too strong."

Constance described well the nightmare experience which cervical cancer or any cancer can become. In her fight against cancer, she took the opportunity to institute changes in her life to better her chances of surviving. Constance modified her diet, her physical activities, and her spiritual life to this end. Despite doing everything she could, her cancer returned in a way that greatly reduced her chances of surviving. About two months after our conversations with Constance, she died from her disease.

In reading these accounts of other women coping with their cervical disease, you may have gained some insight into the universal experience of women dealing with adversity and using their best resources to do what is best for them. In the next chapter we provide additional tools for optimizing your health and information for optimizing your Pap smear.

E I G H T

Obtaining an Optimal
Pap Smear Result

In the preceding pages, we have discussed the implications of an abnormal Pap smear result. We have discussed how the Pap smear is actually a test for tissue changes of the human papillomavirus or HPV, a virus which is both sexually transmitted and is thought to be the causal agent of both precancers and cancers of the cervix. In chapter 3, we focused on interpreting your own Pap smear report. As you recall, this report consists not only of a diagnosis but the important statement of specimen "adequacy." We have tried to emphasize that *not all Pap smears can be read with equal degrees of confidence.* There are extenuating circumstances that can render a Pap smear barely readable or even uninterpretable. These Pap smears are flagged by a "limited" or "unsatisfactory" comment. As we suggested earlier, a "limited" reading may cause you or your clinician to want to repeat a particular Pap test, depending on your clinical circumstances such as previously having a SIL. Of course, an "unsatisfactory" Pap smear must always be repeated.

In this chapter, we will be suggesting ways in which you can reduce the risk that your Pap smear will be "limited" or "unsatisfactory" and optimize your chances of receiving a satisfactory Pap smear result. There are a few surprisingly easy ways to get the most out of your gynecologic exam and Pap test. Instead of waiting to hear that your Pap smear was "limited" or "unsatisfactory," we will suggest ways to avoid those situations that can jeopardize a Pap smear. We will tell you what you *must* tell your clinician so that she can correctly assess your risk for developing cervical cancer and treat you accordingly.

155

As we have learned, because the interpretation of Pap smears is done by people and not by machines, Pap smear diagnoses can be somewhat subjective. Pap smear interpretive skills vary from laboratory to laboratory, as one might expect in a field where so much depends on experience and tight quality control. With this in mind, we will suggest eight questions to ask your healthcare provider about the laboratory reading your Pap smears. In certain specific instances you may even want a second opinion on a Pap smear, a series of Pap smears, or a set of Pap smears and cervical biopsies. We will tell you under what circumstances you may want to consider asking for a second opinion and what your rights are as a patient in this regard. As we stated in the beginning of this book, we feel that your gynecologic health (not to mention your overall health!) must be the joint concern of you and your healthcare provider. In this chapter, we help you help your clinician provide the best gynecologic care possible.

TALKING TO YOUR PROVIDER

Although it may seem old-fashioned in this age of high-tech medical instrumentation, the single best source of information about a patient remains the patient herself. Therefore, it is very important that you discuss any unusual aspects of your reproductive or sexual health with your clinician. Also important is both your past medical and family history.

What does this include? In the case of cervical disease, this certainly includes any history of prior atypical Pap smears, perhaps when you were younger or under the care of another clinician. If you have had prior colposcopies and/or cervical biopsies, your clinician needs to be informed of this and those past reports should be made available to him.

It is an excellent idea to have your records transferred from your old physician's office to your new one whenever you are changing doctors. Many people hesitate to do this, perhaps feeling that a physician or other healthcare practitioner will be insulted if you leave her care. While this may or may not be true, nonetheless it is important that your new clinician has access to information from previous laboratory tests, data from physical exams, and old office notes. You may be surprised to learn that unless you actually request a transfer of your old clinician's office notes, your new clinician will not have access to this information. Transferring your chart is usually just a matter of calling and making the request of office staff. Occasionally you may be required to pay for copies or give a written consent.

If you have had atypical Pap smears, ask specifically that copies of those reports be sent to your new clinician's office. These results may not always be mentioned in your chart and it is important that your new clinician have this information. It is also important for you and your new practitioner to know the circumstances of the atypical results. Was the lab leaning toward a reactive condition or a precancer? Was the Pap smear considered adequate for evaluation, or "satisfactory"? If unsatisfactory or suboptimal, what were the reasons?

Hopefully, a new clinician will take a careful history, including a family history, during your first visit. However, if it doesn't come up, tell your clinician if you have a family history of cancer, especially of the reproductive tract (uterus or endometrial cancer, ovarian cancer, cervical and vulvar or vaginal cancer) in a close female relative (sister, aunt, or mother). While you do not "inherit" cancer in the same way that you inherit your mother's blue eyes, it has been noted that cancer can run in families. Researchers in Sweden have noted this trend in cervical cancer. Your clinician needs to be aware of this piece of your family background.

You also need to tell your practitioner about your lifestyle as it pertains to your cervical cancer risks. She will most likely be aware of your contraceptive choice (for a further discussion of contraception and cancer risk, see chapter 10) but it is also important to let her know if you have had more than one male sexual partner in recent months. Since cervical cancer is, in essence, a sexually transmitted disease, it stands to reason that your risk of contracting the HPV virus with its attendant cancer risks increases with each additional partner. It is also important to provide information about other sexually transmitted diseases you may have had in the past such as gonorrhea, syphilis, or chlamydia. This can indicate a higher risk of HPV and SIL.

This is probably a good place to discuss the all-important doctor-patient relationship. In our opinion, you have won half the battle against cervical cancer if you enjoy a solid relationship with your healthcare provider. A 1999 issue of the *Journal of the American Medical Association* reported on a study of 1,000 patient-doctor conversations and found that nine out of ten patients felt that they had received an insufficient explanation of treatments and tests that had been recommended to them. This may be particularly true when dealing with sexually related medical issues. In our conversations with women, we were surprised to find that this held true for women with cervical problems. Several women stated that they were never told that their HPV infections had been sexually transmitted. We also found that many women find it difficult to initiate conversations with their physicians pertaining to sexuality, even in this era of safe-sex awareness. Conversely, many physicians are unlikely to directly ask their female patients about specific details of their sexual lives, including the number of partners they have. Yet it is this type of information that is critical in assessing your risk of contracting HPV and cervical cancer.

Of course, ideally our healthcare providers are people to whom we can feel free to reveal the most sensitive and confidential information. This entails developing a relationship based on confidence and trust. If you are having great difficulty in sharing sexually related matters with your clinician, perhaps this is a sign that you need to seek out another caregiver with whom you feel more comfortable.

Your relationship with your doctor may not seem very important if you use your physician or other healthcare provider merely as a source of laboratory testing or as a specialist referral. However, if you are not involved in a close doctor-patient relationship, you are cheating yourself of a reliable source of clinical expertise and advice, particularly when something goes wrong. This relationship should be with someone who, in addition to demonstrating sound clinical judgment, is also caring, kind, and a good listener.

Other sorts of information you need to share with your clinician include whether or not you are a smoker since smoking has been demonstrated to increase one's cervical cancer risk. A "compromised" immune state also can lead to an increased risk for developing cancer. This includes both diseases such as HIV infection as well as altered immune states from organ transplantation or cancer chemotherapy. The clinician performing your Pap smear should be aware of any major influences on your health even if you routinely see another physician for your nongynecologic health care.

Last, be sure to let your doctor know about any new and/or worrisome symptoms with your reproductive tract. This would include bleeding or spotting after intercourse, spotting between periods, and pain during intercourse among others. While all of these symptoms are usually caused by innocent conditions, they can also be early signs of malignancy of the female reproductive tract. For example, advanced cancers of the cervix can cause the mucosa or covering of the cervix to become "friable" or bleed easily. This can make itself known to you as bleeding after intercourse. *All new symptoms of the reproductive tract should be taken seriously by you and your physician.*

If you are one of the many women who use a gynecologist as her primary-care physician, be sure that you are also receiving other "standard" health screenings including a breast exam and a rectal exam looking for cancers in these areas. Older women should also be receiving routine mammograms, with the first "baseline" exam by ages thirty-five to forty. The first mammogram is known as the "baseline" because all subsequent exams are compared against it.

SCHEDULING YOUR APPOINTMENT

Since many of the "limited" Pap smears we sign out are due to an abundance of blood on the slide, it makes sense to *not* schedule your Pap smear and exam while you are having your period. Since most gynecologists make their appointments for routine exams many weeks or months in advance, this necessitates either compulsively careful scheduling or extreme good luck.

Mary's gynecologist had an office manager who kept lists of women who cancelled their appointments because of their periods. This office manager would then "swap" appointments so these women could have an appointment after their period was over instead of waiting for the next opening months away. Unfortunately, this is not a common practice and in fact, Mary's gynecologist became busier and a new office manager declined to keep up this laudable practice.

Because it can be very difficult to read a Pap smear accurately if the test is conducted while you are in the midst of your period, whenever possible, try to schedule all your gynecology appointments during your "midcycle," that is, between menstrual periods. The easiest way to do this is to keep track of your cycle on a small calendar in your purse or at work or at home and count two weeks after the first day of your last period. If that day is February 5, for example, and you need to make an appointment for a return visit in six months, you should shoot for August 5 for your next appointment. This may not work if you are very irregular in your cycles or have entered the perimenopausal period of your life and cannot predict your cycles with accuracy.

Should having your period cause you to cancel your appointment? This very much depends on how much you are bleeding. Ideally, you should not be bleeding heavily when your Pap smear is taken. If your flow is very light, for example at the very beginning or end of your period, it probably doesn't matter very much. Also, if your practitioner uses a liquid-based Pap smear test (see chapter 9), the likelihood that your cells will be obscured by blood is lessened, although heavy blood flow will make even those types of tests less than effective.

Additionally, if one or more of your previous Pap smears was "limited," it may make sense to reschedule your appointment at midcycle rather than increase your odds of receiving yet another limited Pap smear. If you are having a repeat Pap smear taken after an atypical or ASCUS Pap smear, it is probably prudent to have your repeat Pap smear taken under the most advantageous conditions possible such as after your period has finished.

It is also a good idea to abstain from sexual intercourse for one or two days prior to your Pap smear. Sperm, lubricants, and contraceptive creams and jellies can be seen on a Pap smear and can occasionally obscure the cells. It is also wise to not douche prior to a gynecologic exam since this can wash away signs of an infection such as an abnormal vaginal discharge.

INFECTIONS

What about receiving a Pap smear during an active vaginal infection or while you are undergoing treatment for an infection? Once again, this very much depends on the severity of your infection, but in general, scheduling a Pap smear during an active infection is a bad idea for at least two reasons.

Like blood from a heavy menstrual period, a large amount of bacteria or yeast organisms can obscure the important cells of a Pap smear and lead to a "limited" reading. Often, it is not the organisms per se, but the abundant inflammatory cells (white blood cells) that arrive on the scene to try and contain the infection that actually cause a Pap smear to be less than fully readable. These white blood cells surround the cells in question and can lie over the cervical cells in large drifts, making it impossible to see the squamous and glandular cells that make up a Pap smear.

Infection and inflammation can have a pronounced effect on cells from the cervix. As we have discussed previously, an infection can cause marked nuclear changes in cervical squamous and glandular cells which are usually correctly interpreted as "reactive" in nature (within the normal range) during a test reading. However, if the changes are severe, they can also be interpreted as "atypical" or even misinterpreted as those of a squamous intraepithelial lesion (SIL) or precancer. Clearly, the ideal situation would be to take a Pap smear at midcycle, when you are free from vaginal or cervical infections.

How long should you wait after a vaginal infection is treated before scheduling a Pap smear? Usually, a three- to four-month waiting period is sufficient for clearing up any reactive changes which are due to an infectious organism. Obviously, a repeat visit to your gynecologist may be called for if your symptoms do not resolve. This is particularly important if you are treating yourself with over-the-counter medications as you might be if you had a yeast infection. Occasionally, symptoms such as itching and a discharge will be caused by noninfectious sources such as an allergic reaction to soaps or detergents. Whatever is causing your symptoms, it is wise to get the condition under control before having a Pap smear.

Which infections are the most likely to cause problems with a Pap smear? In our respective practices as pathologists, we generally see the most problems with yeast infections and with bacterial "vaginosis." Trichomonas infections can also cause a lot of difficulties in reading a Pap smear. A genital herpes infection can also occasionally cause such an extreme degree of reactive changes that cells are interpreted as "atypical."

It is unusual to see the infections that most of us associate with venereal diseases such as syphilis, gonorrhea, and chlamydia, at least in our practices. These infections are still around, however, so you should always engage in safe sexual practices with a condom whenever you have a new partner. As we have mentioned before, and emphasize again here, condoms will not help you avoid being infected with HPV, since it can also be present on male genital skin not covered by a condom. The common vaginal infections we see on a Pap smear are summarized below.

Yeast Infections

Yeast or fungal infections of the female genital tract are extremely common. In fact, most women have probably had one such infection at some point in their lives, although some women seem to be plagued by them. There are particular "states" or physical situations that can make fungal infections more common. Pregnancy, with its many hormonal changes, is one such state. A good environment for fungal infection can be created by using oral antibi-

otics, which kill off "beneficial" bacteria, thereby altering the microenviron-
ment or flora of the vagina in such a way as to make infection likely.

The vast majority of the time, these infections are caused by a common
fungus known as *Candida albicans*. The symptoms are usually pretty easy to
detect and include a thick white discharge most often described as resembling cottage cheese. The discharge often has the odor of bread or yeast.
Itching and irritation of the vulva can be intense. The treatment consists of an
antifungal cream or vaginal suppositories such as Monistat®, which is now
available over-the-counter. A vaginal yeast infection can also be treated with
an oral medication, Diflucan®, which can only be obtained by prescription.
Male partners usually do not need to be treated and there is no need to abstain
from intercourse during treatment.

Trichomonas

A less common infection is *Trichomonas vaginalis* or "trich," which is an
infection by a sexually transmitted microscopic parasite. Women with this
infection complain of both itching and a discharge that may be abundant,
yellow, frothy, and malodorous. The treatment of choice is metronidazole
(Flagyl®). Since a patient's sexual partner is the usual source of the infection,
repeated reinfections may occur unless the partner is treated simultaneously
similarly with metronidazole.

Bacterial Vaginosis

A woman's vagina normally is host to various helpful bacteria, all of which
help to maintain the vaginal environment at a healthy low (acid) pH. On a
Pap smear, these normal bacteria, known as Doderlein bacteria, resemble thin
red crystals. Occasionally they are overgrown by other bacteria that look like
short rods with a dark purple color. These latter bacteria can cover a Pap
smear and make its interpretation very difficult. In the past, these infections
were thought to be due to a single bacteria known as *Gardnerella vaginalis*
or *Hemophilus vaginalis*. We now know that this condition is caused by an
overgrowth of several different bacteria.

Bacterial vaginosis can produce mild itching and a gray liquid discharge
that may be malodorous. However, many women who test positive for these
bacteria do not have any of the accompanying symptoms. This condition is

generally not treated unless the woman complains of symptoms. The treatment of choice is again metronidazole. Other treatments include a vaginal gel (Metrogel®) and a Cleocin® vaginal preparation used at bedtime. Partners do not need to be treated.

"REACTIVE" OR "INFLAMMATORY" CHANGES WITHOUT AN INFECTION

Although a vaginal or cervical infection can cause alarming changes in the cervical cells seen on a Pap smear, the truth is that most Pap smears with reactive changes and abundant inflammation do not have any evidence of an infectious agent. What then is causing the changes? It may be that an infectious organism is causing inflammatory changes but that the organism has either not been picked up and smeared on the slide or the "organism load" (the number of organisms that were caught in the Pap test) is too small for it to be recognized in the Pap smear. However, the more likely explanation is that cervical smears in some women will always harbor some degree of inflammation and "reactive" change for unknown reasons. Perhaps hormonal effects are in play since it is not uncommon for postmenopausal women to have severe inflammation and reactive changes noted on their Pap smears.

Other women may be experiencing the effects of mild reactions to soaps, feminine hygiene sprays, douches, or detergents or even to material in condoms used by their partners. Suffice it to say that some women seem doomed to have Pap smears that are never quite normal but are constantly read as "ASCUS, favor reactive changes" or are limited by inflammation.

Because of the wide overlap in reactive changes and those changes caused by the HPV virus, women in this category need to have close follow-up. This can be extraordinarily nerve-racking and, in fact, this group of women may turn out to be good candidates for the HPV test. If the test was found to be negative, it is likely that the changes seen are due to causes other than the human papillomavirus and are unlikely to be precancers. (The new HPV test is discussed in chapter 9.)

SMEARS WHICH ARE LIMITED BY
AIR-DRYING OR THICKNESS

Occasionally, a "limited" Pap smear will be brought about by factors that have nothing to do with the cells in your cervix or the environment that they are exposed to but instead have everything to do with your clinician's technique in conducting the Pap smear test. A test that is read as "satisfactory for evaluation but limited by smear (or cell) thickness" tells you that from one-half to three-quarters of the slide could not be seen because the cells were clumped together and were too crowded to allow the cytologist to see through them. A successful Pap smear very much depends on your clinician's skill in smearing the cells from your cervix onto the glass slide. If the cells are smeared in a big clump of cells and mucus, it may not be possible to decide definitively whether the cells are normal or abnormal.

Another common reason for a Pap smear being called "limited" has to do with air-drying. A Pap smear's success depends very much on the quality of the staining or "dyeing" of the cells so that the all-important nucleus is seen as a crisp outline with its inner details clearly delineated. The Pap smear stain only works when the cells on a slide have been rapidly "fixed" or sprayed with fixative. Cells that spend even a few extra seconds drying on a glass slide can lead to a Pap smear being read as "limited" due to air-drying. This common problem in slide preparation finds the affected cells blown up to huge proportions and the clear quality of their nuclear detail is lost with the nuclei appearing smudgy and dark. These changes are sometimes flagged on a Pap smear report as "limited due to poor preservation of cells."

However the change is described, it can impede correct interpretation of your Pap smear. If you are receiving repeated Pap smear reports that are limited due to air-drying, your clinician may have better results with a liquid-based Pap test. Since these Pap smears are performed by immediately immersing the cells into fluid, air-drying is not a problem (see chapter 9).

THE REPEAT PAP SMEAR

Your practitioner may have advised you that you will need a repeat Pap smear. Perhaps your Pap smear was read as ASCUS (atypical squamous cells of undetermined significance) and you were advised to obtain a repeat test.

Or perhaps your Pap smear was normal but limited due to an overabundance of inflammation or a lack of endocervical cells and you have a long history of atypical results or even prior diagnoses of SIL or dysplasia. Or maybe you received a diagnosis of LSIL and your clinician has chosen to do repeat Pap smears to see if these changes disappear on their own.

Whatever the reason, the temptation is great to hurry and repeat the Pap smear as soon as possible. The anxiety that accompanies a repeat Pap smear can lead many women to want to try and resolve the uncertainty quickly. As we explained in chapter 4, however, this is usually not the best course of action since even a seemingly gentle scrape of cervical cells can introduce enough trauma (irritation) to cervical tissues so that they respond by showing "reactive" changes. These changes can lead to yet another abnormal Pap smear if the smear is taken too soon. This is particularly important in a Pap smear taken after a cervical biopsy or a cone biopsy since these are particularly traumatic procedures. Although it is emotionally hard to do, it is important to wait a full three to four months before having a Pap smear repeated.

THE CYTOLOGY LABORATORY

As you might expect, the people who interpret your Pap smear are an important part of the process of cervical cancer prevention. Not surprisingly, cytology laboratories are not all the same. Some laboratories are huge private laboratories handling hundreds of thousands of Pap smears a year and employing upward of twenty or more cytotechnologists, while others are small, affiliated with a community hospital, and have a single cytotechnologist reading barely a few thousand Pap smears a year. Some laboratories have pathologists specializing in cytology as their medical directors, while other labs are run by general pathologists who also look at biopsies, do autopsies, and run clinical laboratories.

Laboratories also have different means of communication with their physician-clients. Some will call the clinician for diagnoses of high-grade SIL or cancer and some will fax or flag these diagnoses in some other way. You should be aware of the Pap smear laboratories to which your test may be sent for review.

Listed below are eight questions you can ask your gynecologist about the laboratory handling your Pap smear. Good clinicians are very well informed about the labs that handle their Pap smears and usually have a fairly good idea about which services the laboratory routinely provides. In case the doctor is not sure of the answers to some of these questions, the medical director of the laboratory reading your Pap smears should be readily available to you. You have a right as a patient using the services of the laboratory to have answers to your questions about those services.

EIGHT QUESTIONS TO ASK YOUR DOCTOR ABOUT YOUR CYTOLOGY LABORATORY

1. *How many years have you used the laboratory?* Obviously, the longer your clinician has used the services of the lab, the more experience she will have had with the way the lab handles most of its cases. For example, if she is aware that a lab has diagnosed many of the Pap smears from her practice as "atypical" (a high ASCUS rate), then she may be more likely to discount an ASCUS from that laboratory especially if it was an ASCUS favoring reactive changes. Conversely, if the lab has a low ASCUS rate, she may be more likely to take that diagnosis very seriously. She will also have had the opportunity to check the accuracy of Pap smear readings by performing follow-up biopsies. While occasionally a Pap smear diagnosed as a SIL will be followed by negative biopsies (see chapter 5), this should not be a common occurrence.

2. *How large is the laboratory?* From this question you can get some sense of how many Pap smears the lab reads each year. As discussed in chapter 2, all laboratories in this country must follow government regulations on the numbers of Pap smears individual cytotechnologists can safely examine each day. While there is no established minimum "safe" number of Pap smears a lab should be examining each year, it stands to reason that a laboratory needs to be looking at a sufficient number of specimens in order to be able to do a good job with Pap smear screening. Most of us would not want to have a complicated surgical procedure performed by a surgeon who only did one or two of that type of surgery a year. In much the same way, it is a good idea if the laboratory that screens your Pap smears sees enough smears so that all the cytotechnologists and pathologists can keep up their

diagnostic skills. Cytologists also need to have enough experience with difficult cases. Labs who screen small numbers of Pap smears also may have only one cytotechnologist. This makes it difficult for the cytotechnologist to "share" difficult cases.

3. *Is the medical director board certified in pathology with subspecialty qualifications in cytology?* Board certification in cytology is a one-year added qualification beyond the usual four to five years of training that pathologists receive. This is a year spent learning the fine points of cytologic diagnosis, including Pap smear diagnosis, as well as learning laboratory management and compliance with federal guidelines in gynecologic cytology. Pathologists who have completed fellowships in cytology have had the opportunity to discuss and study many of the problematic areas of Pap smear diagnosis including interpretation of the atypical Pap smear. While many cytology labs have pathologists who are board certified in cytology, this is not true for some smaller labs.

4. *What is the laboratory ASCUS rate and what is the ASCUS/SIL ratio?* The two most important numbers in assessing how your cytology lab is doing are the ASCUS rate and the ASCUS/SIL ratio. The ASCUS rate is simply the percentage of cases that a lab calls "atypical." This number varies with the population screened. In other words, if the lab screens many high-risk patients such as young sexually active college-age women, one would expect that the ASCUS rate would mirror this with a higher rate of atypical Pap smears reflecting the higher rate of HPV infection and SILs. Conversely, if the population screened is mostly middle-aged married women, one would expect the rate to be lower since the rate of precancers is low in this group of women. Despite the differences across various populations and age groups, an ASCUS rate of around 5 percent and below is the number most often quoted in the cytology literature as representing a reasonable ASCUS rate for laboratories. A number that is easier to compare between laboratories is the ASCUS to SIL ratio (ASCUS/SIL). This number adjusts for the different populations of women screened by laboratories. For example, one would expect a lab servicing a "high-risk" population and diagnosing a high number of SIL cases to also have a high number of ASCUS cases. On the other hand, a lab servicing a "low-risk" group of women should have a low number of both SIL and

ASCUS cases. The maximum desirable ASCUS to SIL ratio is often cited in the literature as being from 2.5 to 3.0. In other words, if your lab is calling a SIL diagnosis 1 percent of the time, an ASCUS diagnosis should be made no more than 2.5 to 3.0 percent of the time. Too high of an ASCUS rate indicates that there are too many "false alarms" in that laboratory, most likely from reactive cases being over-interpreted as "atypical." This is potentially very important to you as a patient since you do not want to go through the drill of multiple repeated Pap smears and possibly unnecessary biopsies if the changes on your Pap smear would be interpreted as "normal" but "reactive" by perhaps a more experienced laboratory.

5. *Does the laboratory have available the new technologies of liquid-based Pap smears and HPV testing?* Liquid-based Pap smear techniques are becoming increasingly common depending on the area of the country you live in. They tend to be commonly used in the Northeast but less so in the Southwest. While they have definite advantages, they are expensive and may not be helpful for all women. We will discuss the advantages of this technique in chapter 9. If you and your clinician decide that this is a method that may be useful for you, you need to make sure the laboratory looking at your Pap smear offers this technique since not all labs do. The same can be said for HPV testing, which will either be offered at the laboratory processing your Pap smear or at an independent laboratory used by your clinician. We will also discuss this test in chapter 9.

6. *Does the lab routinely contact the clinician for high-grade or cancer Pap smears?* Most laboratories routinely offer this service. This ensures that you will be contacted as expeditiously as possible should your Pap smear show any serious abnormalities. Occasionally, a Pap smear report diagnosing an HSIL will sit on a clinician's desk for days before being noticed by the office manager or physician. Alerting office personnel by calling or faxing these reports helps to ensure that this crucial information gets to you in as timely a fashion as possible.

7. *Does the lab read cervical biopsies and does it correlate the findings for Pap smears and cervical biopsies?* This is an important function of any laboratory that reads Pap smears. Since the Pap smear is a sampling of cells from your cervix, a biopsy, which consists of a larger portion of cells, is often needed to give an accurate diagnosis of the cervix (see

chapter 4). This is particularly true in the instance of repeated atypical readings or other confusing changes seen on the Pap smear. It is critical that the biopsy and Pap smear diagnoses are "correlated" or compared so that any discrepancies between these two diagnoses can be resolved. In fact, this is such an important task that there are federal guidelines in place to insure that this comparison happens. In many labs, a "correlative statement" will show up on either the Pap smear or biopsy report stating that the two tests were compared and agree with each other. If the biopsy diagnosis does not make sense in light of the Pap smear, the pathologist should comment either on the Pap smear or on the biopsy report as to what she believes is going on in the woman's cervix.

8. *What is the usual turn-around-time (TAT)?* The turn-around-time is the time it takes for the lab to process, read, and report your Pap smear from the time it is received from the doctor. You should expect a TAT of a week or so under normal circumstances, although every lab, even good ones, will occasionally experience times when its TATs are prolonged. If you are waiting many weeks for a Pap smear report either your clinician's office is slow in getting that report to you or the laboratory is having problems handling the volume of Pap smears they are receiving. Rarely, it may mean that your Pap smear was lost. It is worth calling your clinician if you have waited two weeks or more for a diagnosis. Good laboratories will also handle Pap smears as "rush" cases if the clinician requests this service. Usually this is done if the clinician is worried about a cancer in the cervix or in any case where an immediate diagnosis is required. Rush cases generally will generate a diagnosis within one or two days of their arrival at the laboratory.

In general, there are just a few things you need to do to guarantee an optimum Pap smear. Most importantly, you should choose your clinician wisely. He or she should be someone you trust and with whom you are able to discuss your most intimate concerns. In the event that you receive an abnormal Pap smear diagnosis, you will need to rely on their opinion and expertise. Second, you should try as much as possible to schedule your appointment under ideal Pap smear-taking conditions (midcycle, no lubricants or intercourse for several days beforehand, and no known infections of the vagina and cervix). And, as we have just discussed, you should make a few inquiries into the laboratory handling your Pap smear. With all of these things in place, you have done all you can to increase your chances of receiving a satisfactory Pap smear result.

In the next chapter we will discuss some of the newer Pap smear technologies, such as liquid-based Pap tests, automated Pap smear readers, and also HPV testing. While proponents of these new technologies are impressed with their potential uses, we will objectively discuss the cons of these technologies as well as the pros.

N I N E

The New Technologies

A BETTER PAP SMEAR?

*J*ennifer *is a thirty-year-old newlywed who was recently diagnosed with cervical cancer. She has had ASCUS Pap smears in the past but several of them were unsatisfactory or limited for various reasons and she neglected to get a Pap smear for a few years thereafter. She has heard about some of the new advances with Pap smears. Would any of them have helped Jennifer get her cancer diagnosis earlier?*

Mary is a forty-two-year-old woman who has had multiple ASCUS Pap smears over the past five years. She has been diligent about following her doctor's recommendations for treatment and has undergone colposcopy and cervical biopsies twice. No SILs have ever been documented. Mary wonders if she has any options for determining if she has cervical disease other than a trip to her doctor's office for more Pap smears every several months.

An anonymous woman calls the laboratory asking about the availability of "that computer that diagnoses Pap smears." Are Pap smears now being diagnosed by computers? Would such Pap smears be more reliable than those screened by humans?

As in most other areas of medicine, technology in the field of Pap smear analysis is rapidly advancing. From cell collection methods to molecular testing for HPV, virtually all aspects of cervical cancer and precancer detection are undergoing evolution. The goal of these new technologies is, of course, to improve upon the conventional Pap smear. But does the Pap smear really need improving? If so, what are the best methods to accomplish this, and which women will most benefit from these advances?

Throughout this discussion, it is important to keep in mind that the majority of women who are diagnosed with cervical cancer have not had a Pap smear in the past three to five years, if ever. *At the present time, having regular Pap smears is indisputably the single best thing a woman can do to prevent cervical cancer.*

As we have emphasized earlier, however, the Pap smear is not infallible. There are women who religiously have their annual Pap smears yet still end up with cervical cancer. We briefly touched on the problem of false negative Pap smears in chapter 2 when we discussed sources of error in the cytology laboratory. False negative Pap smears are tests diagnosed as normal even though they come from women who have a cervical precancer or, rarely, even cancer. Failure to detect early precancers can result in a woman subsequently developing cervical cancer. Of course, failing to detect cancer can be cata-strophic. The primary goal of these new technologies is the prevention of these false negative Pap smears.

WHY DO FALSE NEGATIVE PAP SMEARS OCCUR?

False negative readings occur for a number of different reasons having to do with almost every aspect of the test. The clinician sampling your cervix at the time of your Pap smear may miss the area containing the SIL so the abnormal cells are never even deposited on the glass slide. This may be due to the prac-titioner's technique or to the fact that the area of the cervix involved was so small that it was difficult to sample. Another reason for having a false nega-tive Pap test is poor fixation at the time the smear is taken so that any abnormal cells present on the slide are difficult to interpret. In addition, your cervical cells may be so thoroughly obscured by inflammation or blood that any abnormalities, even if present, are overlooked. Also, when your slide is examined at the cytology laboratory, the cytotechnologist may inadvertently miss seeing the abnormal cells, for any of the above reasons but also simply due to the strain of a very difficult job and human error.

In recent years, newspaper and magazine articles have emphasized the problem of the false negative Pap smear with horrific accounts of women with negative Pap smears dying of cervical cancer. However, when these "negative" Pap smears were reviewed, they revealed that cancer cells were actually present on the slide. Just how serious is this problem of the falsely negative Pap smear? Should you be concerned that your negative Pap smear is actually harboring abnormal cells? What is the real number of abnormal Pap smears that are "missed" or mistakenly diagnosed as negative?

Not surprisingly, this is a difficult number to accurately estimate. According to several recent reviews, the false negative rate for laboratories across the country ranges from 10 to 30 percent—*that is, of Pap smears coming from women with cervical disease, 10 to 30 percent will be incorrectly called normal.* Note that this does not mean that 10 to 30 percent of *all* Pap smears in a laboratory are incorrectly diagnosed but applies just to those Pap smears that should be diagnosed with a SIL or cancer. These typically make up around 1 to 3 percent of a laboratory's Pap smears. In other words, 10 to 30 percent of 1 to 3 percent of a laboratory's smears or a maximum of .3 percent to .9 percent (less than 1 percent) of a laboratory's total Pap smears may be incorrectly diagnosed as normal when, in fact, there is a SIL or cancer present. These are obviously small numbers but, if you are a woman who is untreated because of a false negative Pap smear (particularly if you have not had regular Pap smear follow-up), for you it may be a huge problem.

Bear in mind that, try as we may to improve upon the Pap test, the false negative problem will never entirely disappear. It is in the nature of medical testing that *not all medical problems will be detected with a screening exam.* This is true whether the test is a mammogram, a fetal ultrasound, or a Pap smear. While the Pap smear is an excellent test for detecting women with cervical precancers and cancers, there will always be a small number of women with cervical disease who will go undetected no matter what type of technology is applied to the test.

As we have repeated elsewhere, this is why it is essential for women to have regular Pap smears. The power of this test lies in its repeated application. But for selected individuals, additional types of testing may be helpful in resolving their Pap smear issues. Let us begin by examining these new technologies, the theories behind them, and other issues such as their availability and cost.

THE NEW PAP SMEAR TECHNOLOGIES

The introduction of new technologies for Pap smears began in the early 1990s, and in the decade since then we have already seen some promising products, several of which are probably already available to you and to your clinician. As you may be aware, the process whereby new medical instrumentation or testing is approved by the government can be long and drawn-out. First, there are years of intensive research and development by the manufacturers followed by a period of testing in laboratories on patient specimens. All of this culminates in a formal evaluation by the Food and Drug Administration (FDA) to meet their requirements for approval. Of course, the final test is that of commercial marketplace acceptance by clinicians and laboratory physicians, as well as medical insurance companies and patients. Insurance companies must agree to accept any new technologies in order to cover their costs while patients may end up footing the bill for some of the newer testing not yet covered by their health insurance.

After some initial scuffling, the dust has settled a bit with regard to which technologies seem to be around for awhile, or at least until something more promising comes along. The three main advances we will discuss in this chapter are (1) liquid-based thin-layer Pap smears, the most well known being the ThinPrep® (developed by Cytyc Corporation of Boxboro, Massachusetts) and AutoCyte® products (developed by TriPath Imaging of Redmond, Washington); (2) computer-assisted Pap smear screening systems as represented by the AutoPap® 300 (TriPath Imaging); and (3) human papillomavirus testing, commercially available as the Digene Hybrid Capture II® test (developed by Digene Corporation of Gaithersburg, Maryland). One heavily advertised technology a few years back was the PapNet computer-based screening but it is no longer commercially available.

Liquid-Based Collection or Thin-Layer Pap Smears

Let's return to Jennifer, with cervical cancer, who opened the chapter. She has had several ASCUS Pap smears, some of which were called unsatisfactory and limited for interpretation. If her ASCUS diagnoses were due, at least in part, to poorly visible and difficult-to-interpret cervical cells, perhaps a technology that helps with cell visibility would have helped her receive an earlier diagnosis of cervical cancer.

Thin-layer Pap smear techniques such as ThinPrep® and AutoCyte® represent a new way to collect and prepare cervical samples for cervical cancer screening. Prior to this "liquid-based" methodology, not much had changed in the way Pap smears were collected and processed since the test was first developed in the 1920s. As you recall, a conventional Pap smear is gathered by gently scraping and brushing your cervix to collect squamous and glandular cells. The cells are then smeared on a glass slide followed by rapid cell fixation with spray fixatives. The thin-layer technique eliminates the smearing and fixation steps, both of which can produce a smear that is difficult to interpret. This may be due to problems in the sample itself such as excess inflammation or difficulties that the clinician may have with the smearing or fixation technique.

In these new methods, instead of smearing your cervical cells on a glass slide, the cells are collected on a small plastic broom that is dropped into a small vial of clear liquid preservative. The liquid immediately preserves the cells which effectively eliminates the problem of air-dried Pap smears since the cells are not given the chance to dry out. The preservative also works to lyse or pop any red blood cells that may have ended up in your specimen so that obscuring blood is less of an issue in this type of specimen. With the thin-layer process, inflammatory cells also tend to present less of a visibility problem since, for the most part, they tend to clump into small groups separate from your cervical cells. All of these qualities of the liquid preservative solution are designed to help increase cell visibility, one of the big issues in Pap smear interpretation. The sealed vial is then sent to the cytology laboratory.

Once received at the cytology laboratory, the cells in the vial are ready to be processed and placed onto a glass slide. Processing begins by placing the specimen into a specialized processor. By using various techniques such as suctioning and filtering, this device draws up the liquid with cervical cells, removes debris, and then evenly deposits the cells on a slide in a small circle (figure 9-1). The cells are placed on the slide with minimal overlap (this is the "thin layer" part of the test) so that each cell may be viewed relatively unobstructed by any other cells. Since a traditional Pap smear that is spread too thickly can also lead to suboptimal or unsatisfactory Pap smears, this technique eliminates that problem as well. The slide is then stained as usual using the Papanicolaou stain. The thin-layer slide is now ready to be screened by a cytotechnologist.

The advantages of this method are obvious. Instead of the usual Pap

Abnormal Pap Smears

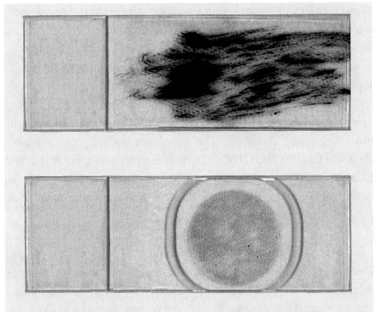

Figure 9-1. Comparison between conventional (top)
and thin-layer (bottom) Pap smears.

smear that may be air-dried, partially covered with blood and inflammatory cells, or thickly smeared, the thin-layer slide consists of a circle of nonoverlapping, well-preserved, and clearly visible cells. But does this method truly increase the ability of the lab to diagnose abnormal cells?

A number of studies have tried to answer this question and report the following: (1) A 1998 review by Austin and Ramzy reported an improved detection of LSILs by 4 percent to 105 percent, although some studies report a decreased detection rate of up to 25 percent. (2) Some investigators have reported an improved detection of HSILs by as much as 100 percent while other investigators have not found an increase in the detection rate of HSILs. (3) Still other studies have reported a lower rate of ASCUS diagnoses, while some laboratories have found a transient increase in ASCUS diagnoses which later levels off. (4) There seem to be fewer unsatisfactory Pap smears and satisfactory-but-limited Pap tests using this new method, although some laboratories have problems finding endocervical cells on this preparation, which can lead to a "limited" reading. In our experience, this sometimes seems to be related to endocervical cells becoming congealed in endocervical mucus. This can make it difficult to see cells within strings of mucus on the slide. (5) Various studies have reported a reduction of the false negative rate; this number also varies considerably depending on the study you are looking at.

As you can see, there are many reported improvements with this liquid-based technique, though those improvements depend heavily on which study is being reported. It is thought by the manufacturers of these methods that the increased detection rates, when present, result from two factors. First, it is hypothesized that sampling is better with a liquid-based technique since nearly all of the cells removed by the spatula and brush will transfer to the liquid, whereas many cells may remain on the collection device when performing a conventional Pap smear, and hence will not be smeared on the slide. Since a liquid-based Pap smear requires that the cells on the collection device be vigorously agitated into a liquid medium, these cells are then available to be processed onto a Pap smear. The cells that would have been "lost" are now present for diagnosis. The second factor has to do with increased visibility of liquid-based preparations. With respect to ASCUS diagnoses, recall that many of these diagnoses result from poorly preserved and poorly visible cells. With the liquid-based method the pathologists viewing your smear can, *in theory*, have an easier time making a firm diagnosis of either "SIL" or "normal" rather than resort to the uncertainty of an ASCUS diagnosis.

We emphasize "in theory" because many of the studies purporting to see improvements in Pap smear diagnoses have been performed under very rigorous conditions with research or academic cytology laboratories. As we observed, there is marked variation in reported improvements in cervical lesion detection in these very carefully conducted studies. The question is whether or not improvements will be seen under the real conditions of a working laboratory, more specifically your laboratory. Not all laboratories will be as successful in decreasing their false negative rates (the number of times that a test is reported as not showing signs of precancer or cancer when the patient is later diagnosed with the disease) as the studies would have us believe. Additionally, some labs will have a problem in *overinterpreting* or *misinterpreting* unfamiliar changes seen on these specimens. This could actually result in more Pap tests being called ASCUS, at least transiently, than perhaps would have happened if they had been taken as conventional Pap smears.

These differences in interpretation occur because the cells seen in a liquid-based preparation are not just clearer but actually look somewhat different from those seen on a conventional Pap smear. This results from the cells floating in solution rather than being smeared on a slide before fixation with alcohol. Most cytotechnologists and cytopathologists have been schooled in conventional Pap smears and derive their experiences from the specific changes seen when sample cells are smeared across a glass slide rather than cells and associated cervical material bobbing around a liquid preservative and then sucked onto a filter.

In fact, the cells in these preparations look different enough that both major manufacturers of liquid-based Pap smear devices conduct "training sessions" so that cytotechnologists and pathologists can learn how to diagnose cervical specimens using these methods. And while it is certainly possible to "relearn" the criteria for various diagnoses on these specimens, depending on the individual cytologist, it can take a while.

If you or your clinician feel that you would be best served by having a "thin-layer" Pap smear, it is probably prudent to make sure that the laboratory looking at your liquid-based Pap test is large enough and experienced enough with this technique to have gone through the "learning curve" these specimens require.

Are there any other disadvantages to this technology? In our opinion, the chief disadvantage probably lies in the increased costs this method introduces. As one would expect with a new technology that requires specialized instrumentation and the use of special collecting devices and preservative vials, there is a substantial increased cost involved with the technique in comparison to the traditional Pap smear. The original (conventional) Pap smear was designed to be a low-cost screening test that could economically screen millions of women. Although liquid-based Pap tests undoubtedly confer some significant advantages in terms of cell visibility, the question is whether the increased cost will benefit you as a patient. If you are in a relatively low-risk category for developing cervical cancer or a cervical cancer precursor, the answer may be no. Women who are in monogamous relationships, who are religious about scheduling their yearly Pap smears, and who have a long history of negative reports may not benefit from a new and more costly technique.

For some women, this technique will be covered by their health insurance plans so that their out-of-pocket costs are minimal or nonexistent. However, for women who do not have this insurance coverage, the cost of the Pap test could add considerably to the costs of their visit to the gynecologist. In the Boston area, for example, if you had to pay for interpretation of a normal liquid-based Pap smear (this does not include your gynecologist's fees), this would cost you about $60. Contrast this to the cost of a normal conventional smear, which is roughly $40 or less.

Because health coverage varies depending on where you live, there may be an uneven distribution across the country of where thin-layer Pap smears are reimbursed and where they are not. In other words, your thin-layer Pap smear may be completely paid for in Texas but not if you live in the neighboring state of New Mexico. If you want a thin-layer Pap smear and you live in an area where there is no reimbursement for the test, expect to pay for this test yourself. Improved reimbursement for thin-layer Pap smears is spreading so it is worth inquiring with your insurance carrier to see if they will cover the cost. Of course, if you are not covered by insurance, you will need to shoulder this additional cost yourself. Again, to decide if this testing is worth it for you, it is important to assess your needs as a patient, the experiences of your clinician, and the experience of the laboratory that will be reading your slide.

Computer-Assisted Pap Smear Screening Devices

This is a good time to think of our anonymous caller mentioned at the start of the chapter and her concerns about "human-read" versus "machine-read" Pap smears. Are there any new techniques in Pap smear screening that utilize the ever-present computer?

Computer-assisted Pap smear screening uses a computer's image-analysis capabilities to screen or prescreen your Pap smear. The computer examines every square millimeter of your Pap smear and has been specifically designed to detect cervical cell abnormalities. The computer, like its live cytotechnologist counterpart, keys in on cell nuclei that are enlarged, dark, or irregular. One computerized device currently on the market is the AutoPap® device (developed by TriPath Imaging of Redmond, Washington). This is an FDA-approved high-speed video microscope with computers to image, interpret, and analyze the cells on a Pap smear.

There are two major ways for a laboratory to use this technology. First, a laboratory can use it to take a second look or "double-check" all Pap smears that their cytotechnologists have diagnosed as normal. In addition, this technology can also be used to perform the government-mandated 10 percent slide rescreening we discussed in chapter 2. Any of these normal Pap smears which look abnormal to the computer will be reviewed again by both a cytotechnologist and a pathologist and a final decision will be made after this third look. Some laboratories may also choose to employ computer imaging to rescreen Pap smears coming from high-risk women, especially women who have had previously abnormal Pap smears. However, the more common practice is for the computer to take a first look at Pap smears ("primary screening"), the job normally done by a cytotechnologist.

With primary screening, the instrument examines all slides from a laboratory. After review, the slides are ranked by the computer from "least abnormal" to "most abnormal." Twenty-five percent of the laboratory's slides are classified as "least abnormal" and then released as "negative" slides. Remember that in the usual situation in which human eyes are screening all slides, characteristically over 90 percent of a lab's slides will be called negative (or normal) with about 10 percent being abnormal. The 75 percent of slides screened by the computer which have not been released as normal will be further screened by a cytotechnologist as is usually done. In other words, the computer has effectively reduced a lab's workload by 25 percent thereby enabling the lab personnel to concentrate on looking at the remaining 75 percent of slides which have the highest likelihood of bearing abnormalities. Many laboratories will also conduct rescreens by a human of any Pap smear coming from a woman with a previous atypical Pap smear, regardless of its ranking by the computer.

Because of the computer's "prescreening" capabilities, the human portion of the Pap test, review of slides by cytotechnologists and pathologists, can now focus specifically on the slides considered at higher risk for abnormalities and use their judgment to determine if cells are normal or abnormal. Remember, the computer is still not "smart" enough to actually diagnose an abnormality. That job is reserved for human eyes and human judgment.

The advantages of this technology are clear. One source of error, the screening error, will be reduced by flagging those slides that require the most vigilant screening. There are now also instruments under development that will combine thin-layer technology with computer-assisted screening.

What are the claims of this technology? According to promotional materials of TriPath Imaging, the manufacturers of the AutoPap® instrument, their own clinical trials claim that the AutoPap® instrument can reduce a laboratory's false negative rate by 33 to 44 percent and decrease false positive readings (Pap smears falsely called abnormal when they really are normal) by 16 percent. They also claim an overall increase of three times the detection rate of LSIL and a fivefold increase in the detection of HSIL.

These are some pretty impressive claims, but like the situation with liquid-based technology, it is unclear how effective this device will be in "real life." We have had discussions with laboratories that currently use this technology and it appears promising. While neither of us currently use computer-assisted screening in our laboratories, we are watching this technology with interest.

What about the disadvantages of this technology? Again, any cost increases need to be considered. The computers are very expensive instruments: in fact, only labs that are processing about thirty thousand Pap smears a year can afford to use this technology. For a large laboratory, the use of computerized screening may increase the cost of a Pap smear by anywhere from three to ten dollars.

Just as with the liquid-based Pap test, the insurance carriers have to be convinced to pay more for this computer-based technology and this, once again, will vary depending on where you live. Will this technology help you, the patient, feel more at ease and confident about the results of your Pap smear? In its present form, computer-based technology is more likely to help a laboratory with its workload than it would help an individual woman concerned about a false negative Pap smear.

On the other hand, could a computer-assisted Pap smear screening device lead to more atypical Pap smears? The manufacturer states that this shouldn't happen. In fact, they claim that a laboratory's ASCUS rate should decrease. It may happen, however, that a pathologist may be reluctant to call a Pap smear normal after a computer has flagged it as belonging to the group considered "most abnormal." From a patient's point of view, this would mean additional follow-up with all its attendant anxieties for a Pap smear that may be very minimally atypical. Once again, a laboratory would need to be experienced in this form of technology before it could derive the most benefit from its use.

Human Papillomavirus Testing

Let's now return to our patient Mary, mentioned at the start of this chapter. She has been plagued by repeated atypical Pap smears, has undergone surgery, and has suffered years of anxiety with no definite diagnosis of a cancer or precancer of her cervix. Since, as we have repeatedly stated throughout this book, the vast majority of cervical cancers are caused by the sexually transmitted human papillomavirus, could a test for HPV help someone like Mary decide if she is truly at-risk for cervical cancer?

In 1999 and 2000, several articles about HPV testing appeared in the *Journal of the American Medical Association*. These caused an intense amount of interest in both the medical community and in the media. In a study performed in the United States at Kaiser Permanente Medical Group, both HPV testing and repeat Pap smears were studied in 1,000 women with ASCUS diagnoses to see which method was better at detecting women with HSIL. HPV testing detected about 89 percent of the women with HSIL which was 13 percent more than were detected by repeat Pap smears. In a study conducted by the National Cancer Institute, 8,000 women from Costa Rica, a country with a high prevalence of cervical cancer, underwent a similar study. HPV testing identified 88 percent of women with HSIL, about 11 percent more than had been detected by repeat Pap smears. Finally, a study from Columbia University of about 1,400 women in South Africa showed similar results and included "self-collected" HPV samples from women. While not as effective as clinician-collected samples for HPV testing, the samples collected by women themselves rivaled a repeat Pap smear in detection of cancers and HSILs.

These articles caused physicians and news reporters alike to ask whether the Pap smear had become obsolete and if testing for HPV should replace the traditional Pap smear.

Before we can answer those questions, it is critical to remember our discussions from chapter 1 regarding the high prevalence of HPV in particular groups of American women compared with the relatively small number of women who end up with serious cervical disease (refer to chapter 1, figure 1-1). In other words, with HPV testing, the concern is not with the false negatives but with *false positives*. In this instance, false positives are seen in women whose HPV tests are positive for HPV but no SILs are detectable by colposcopy and cervical biopsy. This would include the large group of younger sexually active women who are experiencing a transient infection of HPV in their genital tracts but never go on to develop a cervical lesion, much less cervical cancer. If all women with a positive HPV test were told to get additonal follow-up, you can imagine that there would be much anxiety, time, and money spent over nothing since the vast majority of these infections promptly clear up on their own. Is there, then, a sensible use for HPV testing?

In chapter 1 we learned that sexually acquired HPV comes in a number of different subtypes. Some of these viral types are known as low-risk, meaning that they are almost never associated with cancer tissue (although on rare occasions, they can be). These viral types are most often the ones that are associated with genital warts (condylomas). Others are identified as high-risk, which means that they are seen in association with cervical cancer, although not all at the same frequency. Other viral types are "intermediate risk" meaning that although they have been found in association with cervical cancer tissue, they are detected more frequently in high-grade cancer precursors.

The test available today for detecting HPV is the "hybrid capture" (HCII) test from the Digene Corporation. This is a test that looks for the presence of genetic material (DNA) from human papillomaviruses in a sample taken from a woman's cervix. A cervical sample is taken in much the same way it is done for your Pap smear, except it is deposited into a liquid medium. This can be done at the same time as your Pap smear and, in fact, it can be from the same sample used for a liquid-based Pap test. The liquid sample is then sent to the pathology laboratory for HPV testing using the HCII method.

The actual laboratory test combines your cervical sample with a mixture of HPV genetic material to form a hybrid, or a tightly linked match between any DNA from the HPV that might be present in your sample and the standardized HPV material present in the test kit. After a series of detection steps, a brightly colored signal will be produced if HPV is present in your sample. This is detected by a special instrument that reports the results through a computer.

Currently, the HCII tests come in two commercially available types: one searches for a "cocktail" of low-risk subtypes (those most often associated with genital warts) and the second combines both high-risk subtypes as well as those subtypes which are felt to be intermediate risk. Remember that a positive result with the high-risk "cocktail" *does not mean that you are going to develop cancer*. What it does mean is that you have been infected with a viral subtype that has been associated with cancer from laboratory studies. However, many of these subtypes have been found to be associated with LSILs and HSILs *more often* than they have been associated with cancer. With this technology, it is not possible to tell which exact subtype you have been infected with or what your true risks for developing cancer might be.

The above-described HCII test has been approved for use in women. HPV testing in men has been more problematic. Since men can carry the virus in different regions of their genitals, the best way to test for the presence of the virus isn't clear. Although not FDA-approved for this use, HCII may prove of value to the homosexual male population by testing the anal region in those who practice anal sex and are at risk for anal cancer. This is discussed in greater detail in chapter 12.

THE ALTS TRIAL

Let's return to the question of who, if anyone, can benefit from HPV testing. Probably the largest group of women who can potentially gain useful information from this test are women who have been told they have "atypical" or "ASCUS" Pap smears. The idea that HPV analysis may be helpful for women with ASCUS diagnoses has been investigated by a large study funded by the National Cancer Institute. Over five thousand women with either ASCUS or LSIL Pap smear diagnoses were enrolled in this study, which is called the ASCUS Low-Grade Triage Study or ALTS for short. It was designed to explore different treatment options for women who have atypical or LSIL Pap smear diagnoses. In this study, the HCII "high-risk" HPV subtype cocktail was used to determine HPV positivity.

You will recall from chapter 4 that most women with ASCUS diagnoses will go on to have their Pap smears repeated. If the second Pap smear is also read as ASCUS, the woman will most likely go on to colposcopy and possibly cervical biopsy. Women with LSIL diagnoses can elect either to have repeat Pap smears, since 60 to 70 percent of LSILs go away on their own, or head straight to colposcopy. Colposcopy can catch the minority of these women who actually have HSILs. The researchers were interested in finding out if HPV testing could divide women with ASCUS and LSIL diagnoses into two groups: women who could be followed "conservatively" (with repeat Pap smears) because their cervical lesions were not associated with high-risk viruses and women who would be treated "aggressively" (with colposcopy) because they were carrying high-risk viruses. The study did not look at women with diagnoses of HSILs because it is clear that women with that diagnosis need colposcopy and treatment of their lesions.

The ALTS trial has produced results for women with both LSIL and ASCUS Pap smear diagnoses. Published data from this study show that a large percentage of women with LSILs (83 percent) tested positive for high-risk HPV. This large degree of high-risk HPV positivity in women with LSILs suggests that since most women with LSILs will have a positive result, there is no point in doing HPV testing in this group.

The ALTS results also show that about 50 percent of women with ASCUS Pap smear diagnoses were infected by HPV. All of these HPV-positive women then had colposcopy in an attempt to document their cervical lesions by biopsy. Among women ultimately diagnosed with HSIL, HPV testing was 96 percent accurate, compared with a repeat Pap smears accuracy of 85 percent.

It shouldn't surprise us that so many women with ASCUS diagnoses are positive for HPV. From various studies such as those performed by the Kaiser Permanente Medical Groups and Johns Hopkins University, we know that of all women ultimately diagnosed with HSIL on their cervical biopsies, roughly 10 to 40 percent of them will never have a Pap smear with a diagnosis worse than ASCUS. However, in the ALTS study, although approximately one-half of the women with ASCUS were HPV positive, only 11 percent later proved to have an HSIL.

How do these results compare to repeat Pap smears for detecting cervical disease? If you took all women with ASCUS diagnoses and repeated their Pap smears and then sent to colposcopy those women with ASCUS or worse on their repeat smears, you would likely approach the sensitivity of a positive HPV result. Of course, you would need to undergo another Pap smear (requiring another trip to your doctor) rather than going straight to colposcopy with a positive HPV finding. This is an added expense to these additional visits. There is also the concern that some women do not return for repeat Pap smears and are "lost to follow-up." Some of these women may have cancers that go untreated.

In light of these findings, should you be requesting HPV test if you receive an ASCUS diagnosis? Many clinicians and investigators feel the correct answer is yes. A negative HPV result will reassure you that the likelihood of a serious cervical lesion is low. Under these circumstances, some clinicians feel that you could be put back into the pool of "low-risk" women and have your Pap smear repeated in a year's time. This would save you the time and expense of repeated Pap smears, not to mention the anxiety of waiting to find out if your new Pap smear was normal or, once again, atypical. Of course, a second atypical Pap smear usually will buy you an appointment for colposcopy and/or biopsies with all of the attendant headaches of those procedures. If the end result of these procedures is a clean bill of health, you may feel that it would have been preferable to have opted early for an HPV test rather than go through the aggravation of repeated doctor's appointments and procedures. The chances of a woman not returning for essential follow-up would also be reduced.

Some laboratories are now offering so-called reflex testing for HPV. Very simply this means that your physician will ask that an HPV test be performed automatically should you receive an ASCUS diagnosis. This would save you the trouble of a return visit to your clinician as well as save your clinician's office the hassle of calling the lab to request an HPV test when you receive an ASCUS diagnosis. Reflexive HPV testing, however, requires that a cervical sample be available for HPV testing should an ASCUS arise. With thin-layer Pap smears, the same liquid collected for your Pap smear can be used for your HPV test. If your laboratory does not offer thin-layer Pap tests, a separate cervical sample can be collected for future use in special HPV test liquid at the same time as your Pap smear. More guidelines on the use of HPV testing in patients with ASCUS Pap smears will be forthcoming after an upcoming meeting of the American Society of Coloscopy and Cervical Pathology in the fall of 2001.

An important, though infrequently discussed aspect of HPV testing, however, is what do you do if your test is positive but your clinician cannot document a lesion by colposcopy or biopsy? Remember that the majority of women with an ASCUS result and a positive HPV test in the ALTS project did not have serious cervical disease (they were "false positive"). If you recall, the vast majority of sexually active American women will, at one time or another, harbor the HPV virus in their genital tracts, generally in their teens and twenties. This will result in a positive HPV test. For most of these women, the virus is harmless and will disappear on the average within twelve to eighteen months' time. Therefore, if you are in this age group and have an ASCUS diagnosis, you may have a positive HPV test without having cervical disease.

Before agreeing to a test for HPV, *make sure that you can deal with the uncertainty of a positive result if no lesion can be found on your cervix.* This is easier said than done for some women. The idea that they are carrying around a potentially cancer-causing virus in their cervix is more than some women can handle, even if the likelihood is high that this virus will disappear on its own and has not caused any adverse effects (thus far) on their cervical tissue.

In older women (over age thirty-five or so), a positive HPV result may reflect a long-standing persistent infection. These are infections that have a greater likelihood of causing precancers that can progress to cancer. However, it is important to recognize that both researchers and clinicians are assuming that "older" women are in monogamous relationships. In this age of high divorce rates, these assumptions may not be correct. Women who obtain divorces in their thirties and forties may be entering a new period with multiple sexual partners and be newly at-risk for exposure to multiple HPV viruses.

Given all of this, who are the best candidates for this testing? If you have been given a diagnosis of HSIL on your Pap smear, it is clear that you have been exposed to HPV so the test is unnecessary. From the ALTS trial data and other studies, we know that most women with LSILs on their Pap smears will also have HPV in their genital tracts so this information is again not helpful. For women with ASCUS diagnoses, this depends greatly on who you are. Women older than thirty years, particularly postmenopausal women, are probably better subjects for this test. These women are generally out of the age range of the "highly HPV prevalent" younger population who are in their teens and twenties. The presence of HPV in older women may reflect a long-standing infection, one capable of progressing to cancer. Women with multiple and confusing Pap smear and biopsy readings may also benefit from this information as might women who are being followed up after surgery for an HSIL.

The ramifications of an HPV test, whether your results are positive or negative, should be discussed with your clinician. If your follow-up and treatment will not change no matter what the result, it may not make sense to have this information, particularly if you need to pay for it yourself. On the other hand, if a negative result means that you will need no further follow-up, it might potentially save you months of grief and significant amounts of money on more complicated gynecologic procedures if you pay for your healthcare costs out-of-pocket.

COSTS AND AVAILABILITY OF THE HPV TEST

HPV testing is becoming more widely available throughout the country. If the lab which processes your Pap smears does not have HPV testing, your physician should still be able to order it by sending your sample to a reference laboratory or academic center. The test runs about $50 to $60 and is variably covered by insurance.

PROBLEMS WITH THE HPV TEST

How reliable is this test? Will it detect every woman infected by high-risk HPV who is potentially at-risk for cervical cancer? HCII is an excellent test but, like all medical tests, it is not perfect. False negatives may also occur with this test. According to the manufacturer, HCII will detect high-risk HPV in 95 percent of women who have HSIL. This means that at least 5 percent of women with high-risk HPV and SILs will go undetected if the test is done alone.

Another potential problem with the HPV test was brought up earlier. The HCII is a "mix" consisting of a cocktail of different HPV types. In the case of the "high-risk" test, this mix contains a number of viral subtypes that are found most commonly associated with cancer tissue. However, not all of these viral subtypes are equally "aggressive" in their ability to transform cervical tissue into malignancy. For example, HPV 16 appears to be a particularly aggressive subtype while some of the other subtypes appear to be less so and are nonetheless frequently found in association with precancers, both LSIL and HSIL. So just knowing that you are positive for "high-risk" virus by the HCII test does not tell you the complete story. You may be infected by a viral subtype that has only occasionally been found to be associated with cervical cancer. Conversely, you may be harboring a viral type that has been found in cervical cancers at a much higher frequency. There are tests for specific viral types but these tests are usually only done in research or academic settings and are not generally available for clinical use. These types of tests are very time and labor intensive and are not amenable to routine clinical testing. Your clinician would need to specially request this type of test (PCR-Southern blot analysis).

Of course the biggest problem with HPV testing is the high likelihood of false positive results. Depending on your age and life situation, there is a good chance of receiving a positive result that is not reflective of cervical disease. We have discussed this issue above.

HPV TESTING IN DEVELOPING COUNTRIES

Although HPV testing is not meant as a primary screening method, there are some instances where primary screening for cervical cancer may best be done using HPV testing. By this we mean using HPV testing either alone or along with Pap smears as a first-line diagnostic tool. In developing countries, where the prevalence of cervical cancer is high and the availability of Pap smears is low, primary HPV testing may make a lot of sense. This is simply because widely available and easily accessible cervical cancer screening by Pap smears is usually not available for a large part of the female population. Cytology laboratories and certified cytotechnologists are a rarity. In these countries there are many women with cervical precancers who are never diagnosed or treated and predictably go on to develop cervical cancers.

In such countries, a woman may have a pelvic examination and Pap smear only once in her life. This one examination may be the only chance to diagnose and treat cervical disease. In reality, it is easier to teach a healthcare worker to perform and interpret an HPV test result than it would be to teach noncytologists the difficult art of Pap smear interpretation. In these countries, it may be lifesaving to use a test for HPV as a primary screening technique in order to identify women who are infected by high-risk HPV subtypes and hence require follow-up to assess for cervical cancer.

NEW PAP SMEAR TECHNOLOGIES: WILL THEY HELP YOU?

What technologies are most likely to help you with your abnormal Pap smears? Again, we emphasize that the answer to this question very much depends on who you are (your age and other characteristics about you), preferences of your clinician, and characteristics of the lab used by your clinician for Pap smear screening. If the lab to which your clinician is sending her Pap smears does not provide a liquid-based Pap smear option, then you will not be able to have the lab perform that test on your Pap smear. Laboratories that do not offer these new technologies usually can send your specimen to other labs that do.

Also, as directors of cytology laboratories, we would like to point out that some of these new technologies will be more attractive to a clinician if the lab currently handling her Pap smears is not doing such a great job with them! In other words, if a lab is calling many of its Pap smears ASCUS when a healthy proportion of them are probably really "reactive," then HPV testing may be useful in determining which of those Pap smears are more likely to represent significant disease. On the other hand, if the lab has a low ASCUS rate and only calls Pap smears that are "truly" atypical ASCUS, then HPV information may be less useful for the majority of women who are serviced by that lab.

Again we must reiterate that the most important thing a woman can do to protect herself from cervical cancer is to get regular Pap smears. The Pap smear is still the cornerstone of cervical cancer prevention in this country. Medical economists (scientists who look at costs relative to benefits in medicine) state that the most cost-effective way to prevent cervical cancer is to ensure that every woman gets regular Pap smears. This is in contrast to spending huge amounts of money on the development of expensive technologies to make the Pap smear incrementally better.

We wholeheartedly agree that all women need access to routine Pap smear screening. However, as professionals in this field, we are also excited about some of the newer options available to women through our laboratories and we recognize that some of these options may prove to be lifesaving in countries that do not have access to routine Pap smear screening. All of the various technologies discussed above have something to offer by way of improving the current status of screening for cervical cancer in this country and, we hope, throughout the world.

In the next chapter we focus on features of your lifestyle and how they pertain to cervical cancer prevention. As we will discuss, this is an area of somewhat sketchy research. However, there does exist evidence that you may be able to minimize the possibility of serious cervical disease by attending to certain aspects of your everyday life.

T E N

Lifestyle and Cervical Cancer Prevention

One of the great unknowns in cervical cancer research has to do with why relatively few women go on to develop the disease despite the large number who become infected by HPV. Remember that while a cervical infection with HPV is necessary for the formation of cervical cancer, only a very small percentage of all women with HPV infections actually go on to develop cervical precancers or cancer. What is it about that small percentage of women that allows this process of cervical cancer formation to move forward?

We have stated in chapter 1 that poorly understood immune differences and possibly some hormonal factors are currently thought to cause an HPV infection to regress in one woman but develop into a cervical lesion in another woman. Many of these differences undoubtedly have to do with the way our individual immune systems function, which may be genetically based. This might explain at least some of the increased susceptibility to cervical cancer that we see with different ethnic groups such as black, Hispanic, and Native American women. There also seems to be a minor "hereditary" factor so that your chances of developing cervical lesions are increased if your mother had SILs or cervical cancer and if you have been exposed to HPV.

Clearly, there is not much that we can do about our genetic or ethnic backgrounds, but what about the things that we *can* change about our lives, such as nutrition or stress control? It is currently very fashionable to speak about improving immune function with various diets or exercise regimens, and there are many popular books on this topic. But is there any truth to these claims? Is there an optimum cancer prevention lifestyle and if so, are there any data specific to cervical cancer prevention?

Some of the women with cervical abnormalities with whom we spoke had also thought about these issues. One woman who had a cone biopsy for HSIL said that the pain she suffered after her procedure really made her question her frenetic lifestyle. She wondered if there was anything about her life that had weakened her immune system and predisposed her to developing a cervical lesion. She used the opportunity to examine various facets of her life including her diet and her approach to getting sufficient rest.

While we applaud any woman who uses a diagnosis of a cervical abnormality to examine her life and then decide to make healthy choices, we must emphasize that research in the area of cancer prevention and lifestyle is, at best, "soft." Unlike some of the more rigorous studies on the association of HPV with cancer, the studies that look at correlations between nutrition and other factors in cervical cancer prevention tend to be less definitive and should be interpreted cautiously. This type of study is notoriously difficult to design and execute since there are so many variables for which to account. For example, women who tend to eat more healthful diets also tend to visit their doctors more often. They also tend to prescribe to other healthful habits such as avoidance of drugs and cigarettes.

While adherence to a "cancer prevention lifestyle" is probably not a bad thing for most of us, keep in mind that the steps from HPV infection to the development of precancers and cancers are poorly understood and complex. It is unlikely that a single simple maneuver such as taking vitamins will confer absolute protection from cervical cancer. Despite this, it is also true that most of the suggestions coming out of this type of research tend to be generally good for overall health. In this chapter, we will discuss some of the current thinking with regard to cervical cancer risk and lifestyle factors.

YOUR SEXUAL LIFESTYLE

The single most significant factor in whether or not a woman will develop cervical cancer is whether or not she has been exposed to the sexually transmitted human papillomavirus. Since information about this virus is not widely known, many women we spoke to were shocked to find out that the precancerous and cancerous changes that a Pap smear looks for are actually due to the effects of a sexually transmitted virus. Some women were deeply embarrassed that they were now having serious medical problems as a result of a past sexual relationship. Other women found it difficult to psychologically process their "venereal infection" since they did not see themselves as being promiscuous.

As we have stated numerous times throughout this book, cervical precancers and cancer are essentially sexually transmitted diseases resulting from infection by the human papillomavirus which is transmitted during a sexual encounter. If you have never had a sexual relationship with a man, you are at very low, probably zero risk for HPV infection and cervical disease. Remember that intercourse is *not* required for the virus to pass from an infected man to a woman. The virus lives very happily in secretions and on the surface of the scrotum and penis and is easily transferred by genital to genital contact. So being a virgin *does not* protect you from an HPV infection.

By the same token, lesbians are at risk for HPV infection and cervical cancer largely to the extent of any previous male partners. It is known that a large percentage of lesbians have had prior male partners. Transmission of HPV between women is thought to be a rare event although theoretically possible.

If you are like the women we spoke with who were embarrassed at the sexually transmitted nature of their cervical disease, keep in mind some important statistics from the first chapter. Somewhere around 80 percent of sexually active young women at some time will harbor HPV in their cervixes, most often transiently. If embarrassment is the correct response to an HPV infection, then there should be a lot of embarrassed women (and men) in the United States.

Although the majority of sexually active women will have an HPV infection, keep in mind that your chances of both having an infection and then going on to develop a cervical lesion because of that infection increases with the more male sexual partners that you have. This is because multiple HPV types infect the human genital tract and you are increasing the chances of being infected with more than one type of HPV as you have sex with more partners, some of whom may also be infected with more than one HPV type. Therefore, even if your body is able to "clear" an HPV virus (or viruses) from your current partner, there is no guarantee that you will be able to mount the same vigorous immune response to another partner's possibly different set of HPV types. It stands to reason that the more partners you have, the higher the likelihood of developing cervical disease (not to mention other sexually transmitted diseases).

This assumption is confirmed by a study at the University of Michigan School of Public Health which looked at the issue of multiple partners. It found that there was a strong association between the number of sexual partners a woman had and her chances of developing a sexually transmitted infection. Specifically, college women with five or more partners were eight times more likely to have an STD than those with only one partner. If you tend to have a lot of sexual partners, you might want to think about slowing down and becoming more discriminating. Between the human immunodeficiency virus (HIV), HPV, hepatitis, and the usual types of STDs, such as chlamydia, gonorrhea, and syphilis, there are some serious diseases that can befall you by indulging in indiscriminate sexual behaviors. This aspect of your lifestyle deserves careful thought.

TEENS AND HPV RISK

If you are a teen reading this book, the mother of a young teen, or a healthcare professional or educator who works with teenagers, recall that these young women are at particular risk for the development of an HPV-related lesion. As we discussed in chapter 3, the maturing female cervix is undergoing changes that make precancerous lesions with HPV infection more likely. Young teens are much less likely to have transient and harmless HPV infections.

Teens are also more likely to be poorly informed about HPV, cervical cancer, and Pap smears. In a study conducted at the University of New Mexico in 1999, while 44 percent of the teenage girls surveyed were sexually active, only 11 percent knew why a Pap smear is performed. In another study from Canada, 87 percent of the teenagers surveyed had never heard about HPV.

It is difficult to advise abstinence these days since we are surrounded with sexual imagery from television to advertisements at the bus stop. Abstinence, however, is a good idea for young teens under the age of fifteen purely from a cervical cancer prevention standpoint. Young teens should obviously be provided with information on the prevention of sexually transmitted diseases through safe sex and pregnancy prevention with birth control. Mere recommendations for safe sex through condom use, however, simply will not prevent the spread of HPV. Information about HPV and cervical cancer needs to be included in these conversations. As with any discussions with teens, there is the important goal of keeping communication lines open and not alienating them by resorting to scare tactics. However, from a cancer prevention point of view, young teens should not be having sex.

CIGARETTE SMOKING

A woman can add increased susceptibility to cervical cancer to the long list of reasons why she should quit or never start smoking. In studies from the National Cancer Institute and the Karolinska Institute in Sweden, this increased risk is estimated to be at least two times greater than that seen in nonsmokers. There appear to be some subtle interactions between HPV-infected cervical cells and substances found in cigarette smoke that promote the development of cervical cancer. Scientists in New York have identified cancer-causing substances called "nitrosamines" present in cigarette smoke that are also detectable in cervical mucus.

There is a long list of components found in cigarette smoke and several are frank carcinogens (cancer-causing compounds) while many others are mutagens (compounds which cause DNA damage in cells under experimental conditions). The link between cigarette smoking and lung cancer is extremely well established with the carcinogens in smoke acting directly on the tissues with which they come in contact. Other types of malignancies smokers are at an increased risk of contracting include cancers of the mouth, throat, windpipe, esophagus, pancreas, bladder, and possibly the breast. Cigarette smokers are also more likely to develop respiratory diseases such as emphysema and heart disease. Smoking in women can also induce earlier menopause which further increases the risk of developing heart disease. Early menopause also can lead to osteoporosis or thinning bones.

Aside from increasing a woman's risk of cervical cancer, there are other excellent reasons to quit smoking. These include the damage to children, starting from exposure during a woman's pregnancy which can lead to the risk of low birth weight. Later exposure after birth increases a child's risk of serious respiratory problems such as asthma and allergies. More and more damaging information is accumulating on the role of secondhand smoke in promoting cancer (particularly lung cancer) in innocent bystanders inhaling someone else's smoke.

This discussion is in no way intended to minimize the difficulty in quitting such a highly addictive habit. If you are a woman who has tried to quit but has failed using standard therapies, it is worth taking a second or even third or fourth look at quitting smoking. Recent studies indicate that there seem to be sex differences in which strategies are the most effective for long-term smoking cessation in women compared with men. For example, nicotine replacement with patches or gum is usually the first line of therapy but this is often less effective with women.

If you are a woman who wants to quit smoking, there are currently many avenues to help you reach your goal. Aside from the standard nicotine replacements, Zyban® is a prescription antidepressant that has shown promise. If the standard therapies do not work, sometimes various combinations of nicotine replacement together with Zyban® may do the trick. Anecdotally, nontraditional alternatives such as hypnosis or acupuncture may also work with some women. The American Cancer Society is an excellent resource for information on different methods to quit smoking. A phone call to your local chapter may help get you started. It is well worth whatever effort you need to put into this endeavor.

CERVICAL CANCER AND CONTRACEPTION

Your risk for developing cervical abnormalities may also be affected by your contraceptive choice. In several studies from the 1980s and 1990s, such as the one by the National Cancer Institute, women on oral contraceptives seemed to have a higher risk for the development of cervical cancer. This is thought to result from some interaction of the hormones with HPV-infected cervical tissue. The association is not a huge one but it does seem to stand up to the scrutiny of more than one study. It must be stated that this association is not universally accepted and some scientists, such as those at Johns Hopkins University, feel that definite conclusions cannot be drawn based on the available data.

Should you stop taking the Pill because of a possible association between oral contraceptives and cervical cancer? Probably not. If oral contraceptives are your contraceptive method of choice, there were undoubtedly many excellent reasons that you have chosen it. One advantage to oral contraceptives is that they appear to be protective against another female cancer, that of ovarian cancer. Just keep in mind the potential association with cervical disease, and never miss a Pap smear.

NUTRITION

It has been known for some time that certain types of diets, in particular those rich in fruits and vegetables, seem to confer a "cancer protective" effect. Vegetarians tend to get certain types of cancers less frequently. From these observations, however, it has not been possible to differentiate clearly whether this cancer protective effect is due to the actual ingestion of plant foods or whether it is due to the fact that vegetarians do not eat meat. Lately, according to a review by the American Cancer Society on micronutrients contained in plant foods, it seems probable that the protective effects of eating vegetables is due to one or more components of the fruits and vegetables themselves.

Much recent research has focused on chemical substances known as *antioxidants* contained in foods such as fruits and vegetables. Examples of antioxidants include vitamins E, C, and A, as well as beta-carotene and pigmented carotenoids. These substances have the effect of preventing damage to a cell's DNA. This is critical for halting a cell's progression toward malignancy since DNA damage is the first step in this process. Nature has actually made it quite simple to choose foods rich in antioxidants since these substances are contained within fruit and vegetable pigments. So choosing brightly colored fruits and vegetables such as red peppers, plums, berries, dark leafy greens, tomatoes, and pumpkins will guarantee that you are taking in good doses of these important chemicals.

What about plant foods in pill form for those among us who are not vegetable lovers? Our advice is to work hard to develop a fondness for plant foods since it is not known if "vegetables in a pill" offer the same protection against cancer as their fresh produce counterparts. At the very least, they will not provide you with the healthy fiber found in fruits and vegetables.

It is actually not very difficult to disguise vegetables and fruits within soups, breads, or desserts, especially if you are a fussy eater or have a partner or children who balk at too many green things on their plates. We offer several excellent cookbooks for plant foods in our Appendix B.

As far as traditional vitamin supplements are concerned, most nutrition experts and physicians are in agreement that a standard multivitamin pill is probably good nutritional insurance. Many researchers and clinicians alike are also recommending supplemental vitamin E, up to 400 IU (international units) daily, since this vitamin is very difficult to get through dietary means. Vitamin E may confer both a cancer-reducing as well as a heart-protective effect. Folic acid is also an important nutrient for women since it protects against several devastating birth defects and may also protect against heart disease and cancer. You should make sure that your multivitamin contains folic acid. Natural sources of folic acid include orange juice, beans, and leafy green vegetables.

Do any of the above recommendations hold specifically for cervical cancer or SIL? Research in this area offers inconsistent results. According to Dr. Walter Willet, professor of Epidemiology and Nutrition and chairman of the Department of Nutrition, Harvard School of Public Health, he is "not aware of any convincing data that antioxidants, folic acid, vitamin C, or vitamin A will reverse abnormal cervical cytology." As we mentioned in the beginning of this chapter, it can be exceedingly difficult to figure out the precise effects of a particular vitamin or nutrient (vitamin A, for example) while controlling for all other "confounding" factors such as smoking and sexual habits. Also keep in mind that reliable HPV testing is a relatively recent advance so that earlier studies were not able to use positive or negative HPV results in looking for the protective effects of various nutrients.

As summarized in a recent issue of *Alternative Therapies in Women's Health*, studies of cervical disease and diet, for the most part, have shown an inverse association between the risk of cervical cancer and dietary intake of dark green and yellow vegetables, beta-carotene, and vitamins C and E. In other words, the higher the intake of these foods and nutrients, the less chance for development of cervical disease. These types of studies are "observational studies" since they are based on trying to make a conclusion by looking for correlations between a measured variable such as a nutrient and an end result such as cervical precancers or cancer.

The studies which have looked at using nutrients as "medicines" in "interventional studies" have been less successful in substantiating the cancer preventative role that nutrients can play. For example, a multicenter trial in the Netherlands showed no effect of beta-carotene on SIL regression. Trials have been performed on folic acid, beta-carotene, vitamin C, and topical retinoic acid (a vitamin A derivative). The results from these studies seem to indicate that only the retinoic acid applied to the cervix showed any promise of causing cervical lesions to regress. Since retinoic acid has the potential to cause birth defects, women would be wise to await further studies about this nutrient.

For the time being, as we await the research on cervical cancer and nutrients to sort itself out, it seems to make good health sense to increase your intake of fruits and vegetables, with the official USDA recommendation being five fruits and vegetables a day. This recommendation is probably a little on the low side and we could all benefit from eating more plant foods.

OPTIMIZE YOUR IMMUNE SYSTEM

A healthy, well-functioning immune system is absolutely essential to your overall health and well-being. It is your immune system that prevents potential damage from foreign substances such as microorganisms and carcinogens. It is also responsible for getting rid of HPV before it can cause precancerous and cancerous changes in your cervix.

Your immune system consists of your tonsils, spleen, bone marrow, and lymph nodes as well as specialized cells in other tissues such as your intestines and lungs. These tissues produce and circulate cells whose job is to recognize foreign substances and protect you from their ill effects.

We all know that a properly functioning immune system acts to fight infections by microorganisms. There is also growing evidence that your immune system has a role in fighting or preventing cancer by recognition and destruction of cells in your body that have undergone cancerous mutations due to exposure to carcinogens, free radicals, or other events. This is evident in individuals with impaired immune systems who are at a higher risk for cancer. Beyond this fact, can people with well-functioning immune systems lower their cancer risk by boosting their immune systems? The answer is not at all clear although some studies offer tantalizing suggestions that this may be the case.

Most investigators would likely agree, however, that it is wise to limit your exposure to harmful chemicals such as pesticides, herbicides, and cleaning and other solvents and radiation such as unnecessary X rays. We still don't completely understand the damage to cells that can occur from exposure to a variety of chemicals, damage that possibly may result in cancer-causing mutations. These can also theoretically stress your immune system and, if prolonged, could result in your immune system not functioning at its best, thereby increasing your susceptibility to cancer, among other diseases. If you have an occupation or indulge in hobbies where you are exposed to solvents or other chemicals, make sure that you are following all of the manufacturer's recommendations in terms of not breathing fumes for an extended time.

Another area of controversy has to do with the effect of emotional stress on your immune functioning. We all know of instances when we sometimes become ill after marked emotional stress in our lives, whether at work, school, or in social relationships. It is a difficult area for scientists to document but there is an undeniable association between the mind and the body. It seems our immune systems can often be the victim of too much stress. Some writers such as Drs. Andrew Weil and Elinor Levy have speculated that chronic stress can depress the immune system in ways that render us more susceptible to cancer. Whether this is in fact true or not, chronic stress is an unpleasant backdrop to our lives and we heartily endorse whatever methods can be found to help relieve it (as long as this does not include smoking, gobbling cheeseburgers, and having sex with multiple men!).

Ways to reduce stress are many and lend themselves to being individualized for what works for you. Many women find meditation a valuable way to calm the mind and gather resources to face our often hectic and stressful lives. Yoga is an excellent way to incorporate mental relaxation, flexibility, and balance. Some of the more vigorous varieties, such as Astanga or "power" yoga, even provide an excellent strength workout. Yoga can be of particular benefit as we age, since balance and flexibility are crucial for being able to stay independent. A nice massage or bodywork of some kind is also an excellent outlet for mental stress, which can manifest itself in tight muscles. Aerobic exercise is the trick many women use to combat stress in their lives. Aerobic exercise for about half an hour four to five times a week will not only be beneficial for your cardiovascular health but will keep your bones and muscles fit, your gastrointestinal tract running smoothly, and calm your mind. Strength training with weights is also a wonderful stress-reliever while giving you the added benefit of looking and feeling strong.

Do not underestimate the importance of friends in your life. A good friend can make the darkest moments much more tolerable. A great friend can make you laugh about them. Women have traditionally reached out to each other during times of crisis because this is a stress-reducing maneuver that works. It is recommended that you "mix it up." In other words, demonstrate diversity in your choices of stress-busters. Make room in your life for a combination of exercise, meditation, massage, and a long chat with a good friend.

The above discussion points out how much we have yet to learn about HPV infection, cervical cancer, and how women live their lives. If you are a woman with cervical disease, now is the time to examine your lifestyle choices: your sexual behavior, your diet, and your choice of stress reducers. And don't forget to schedule regular Pap smears! More than ever, we women have the power to shape our own futures and enjoy a healthy, cancer-free old age.

Our discussion up to this point brings us to the present state of cervical cancer detection. A number of new avenues for advancing our knowledge are quietly developing in the wings of medical research. The next chapter discusses some of these new frontiers and their promise of improved prevention, detection, and treatment of SILs and ultimately cervical cancer.

ELEVEN

New Directions in Cervical Cancer Prevention

T his book has focused on the most current information about abnormal Pap smears. Here we will look beyond the present to the near future and see what Pap smear-related developments are in the offing. While some of these developments may have implications for you, others may only be of benefit to the next generation of young women to face abnormal Pap smears, which includes our daughters and granddaughters.

PHARMACOLOGIC APPROACHES TO HPV

With Aldara® (Imiquimod) cream for the external treatment of genital warts (or condylomas), we have entered a new era of medical therapy for diseases caused by HPV. These warts are the fleshy growths, caused by lower-risk strains of the HPV virus, which appear on the external genitals and around the anus of men and women. Previous treatments for these lesions included cryotherapy (freezing), laser surgery, and very harsh medications. It is unclear exactly how Aldara® works, however, it is thought that it has a modifying effect on a patient's immune response. The cream does not appear to have any direct antiviral effects.

In a clinical study sponsored by the 3M Corporation, the drug company that manufactures Aldara®, 50 percent of the subjects experienced complete clearance of their genital warts in around ten weeks. In contrast to other treatments, side effects were generally limited to redness and skin peeling. The suggested use of this cream is a three-times-weekly application at bedtime with the cream washed off in the morning.

While this product is strictly for use with external genital warts and not for treatment of cervical SILs or precancerous lesions, the concept appears promising for treatment of vaginal and cervical precancers. If such a medication is shown to be effective against cervical SILs, it may allow women to avoid pain and later scarring, both of which are problems with the surgical approaches to treatment of SILs.

To date there have been no clinical trials of Aldara® for this purpose and the therapies described in chapter 4 are the standard of care for SILs. Though it is premature to recommend this type of therapy for SILs, there is intense interest in its application.

OPTICAL DEVICES FOR CERVICAL CANCER SCREENING

Some very different technologies are being explored in the early detection of precancers. These involve the ability to look at the cervix using special optical devices and determine without a microscope the presence of HPV infection and cervical disease. Some of the different optical devices being explored include infrared, ultraviolet, and fluorescent instruments, to name a few. These special optical instruments would be present in the colposcope your doctor uses to inspect your cervix. These are all in very early stages of development and it is too soon to report on their potential.

If these techniques bear fruit, they may provide a way of looking at a woman's cervix to acquire a "real time" estimation of her HPV status and any HPV disease. A complete evaluation could be done in one doctor's visit and provide an immediate, on-the-spot answer about a woman's HPV status and the presence of SIL. Conceivably a woman could be diagnosed and also treated for her lesion at the same visit. This approach has the potential to eliminate multiple doctors' appointments and many months of anxious waiting that we often see with today's treatment of atypical Pap smears. This approach would also be of great value in developing countries where Pap smear screening for cervical cancer is limited. In this way a woman may receive a Pap smear, be closely examined for cervical disease, and treated in just one visit.

NOVEL CELLULAR "MARKERS" FOR CERVICAL DISEASE

Since only a small percentage of all HPV infections actually lead to precancers, it would be helpful if we could somehow identify those specific infections before they result in precancerous changes. Recent research indicates that this may soon be possible. A group of investigators at the University of Heidelberg in Germany have found that a patient's own cervical cells increase the amount of a specific protein called p16INK4a when the cell is "transformed" by HPV. They claim that by monitoring the increase of this protein this will tell us which cells are not just infected by HPV but will go on to develop precancerous changes.

By developing techniques to recognize this protein in a patient's Pap smear sample, it will be possible to identify which patients are at-risk for developing SILs. Research on using information about the p16INK4a gene is ongoing in several laboratories abroad and at the National Cancer Institute in this country.

HPV VACCINE DEVELOPMENT

The treatment of HPV lesions detected by Pap smear is currently accomplished by physically removing lesions by electrocautery, scalpel, laser, or cryotherapy. These treatments have had a tremendous impact on reducing the incidence of cervical cancer in developed countries. They are, however, also very costly and depend on well-organized healthcare delivery systems. These systems are not present in developing countries, where the incidence of cervical cancer makes it the number one or two malignancy found among women.

In the United States alone, somewhere between four and five billion dollars a year is spent on cervical cancer screening and treatment. Despite this huge financial outlay, an unacceptably high number of women in this country still die from cervical cancer. Is there a more cost-effective way to address this problem? Is there some way to protect all women from cervical cancer, even women from traditionally underserved parts of the country? We also need to think globally and consider solutions that could impact the incidence of HPV disease and cervical cancer where it is most needed, in developing countries with limited monetary and healthcare resources.

Treatment and removal of HPV lesions by our standard treatments does not mean that the virus has been eliminated from a man or woman's body. HPV can still be present in a treated person's tissues, perhaps ready to infect other partners or to form HPV lesions at a later time. The current medical approach to HPV, consisting of Pap smear screening and treatment of discovered HPV lesions, really has no way of making an impact on the widespread prevalence of the infection. To really work on preventing cervical cancer on a worldwide basis another approach to HPV is clearly needed. This may well be a vaccine for HPV that utilizes a person's own immune system to fight the virus, potentially prevent infection, and possibly reduce the absolute incidence of the infection.

The importance of an individual's immune system in handling an HPV infection has been stressed numerous times throughout our discussion. Much of this immune response is unfortunately still a mystery. Although other factors are likely involved, we know that a woman's immune response to HPV is very important in preventing the progression of HPV infection to precancerous and then to cancerous disease.

We have seen tremendous successes in the past in reducing the deaths from other infectious diseases by immunizations. Smallpox, polio, and hepatitis B are just some examples of other viral infections that have been controlled by the widespread use of immunizations. At present, there are determined efforts to accomplish the same success with genital HPV infections using a vaccine against the virus.

Development of vaccines in general can be a complicated process. Traditional vaccines contain some particle of a virus that is enough like the whole virus to stimulate a person's immune system to produce antibodies powerful enough to kill the virus. In other words, a vaccine essentially tricks the body into thinking it is being infected and the body responds by making lethal antibodies against the virus. Specialized immune cells remember how to make these specific antibodies after the vaccine has prompted their initial production. If at a later date the virus actually does infect you, antibodies will be produced and released that kill the virus before it can do any harm.

A complicating factor with an HPV vaccine is the fact that there are a number of HPV types that cause genital infections. For any HPV vaccine to be effective, it must contain parts of all the major HPV types that are important in cervical cancer development: the major high-risk HPV types such as HPV 16, 18, 31, and 45 for a start. A vaccine that covers multiple HPV types is known as a "polyvalent or multivalent vaccine" as compared with a "monovalent vaccine" that covers just one HPV type, such as HPV 16.

To further complicate the issue, we now know that HPV 16 in North America is different from HPV 16 in Asia, Africa, and South America (and those three are also different from each other!). This means that different HPV vaccines may have to be developed for different parts of the world. We do need to keep a global approach in mind since it is still the developing countries where cervical cancer continues to be rampant and where there are limited resources, financial and medical, for large-scale Pap smear screening. Also, the world is much smaller than it used to be and a problem in one part of the world, such as antibiotic-resistant strains of tuberculosis in Asia, can end up on the streets of New York or any other major city.

Given that designing an HPV vaccine will certainly have its challenges, what is currently happening with vaccine development? There are two approaches presently being pursued for an HPV vaccine. The first is for therapeutic or treatment use in women who already have cervical cancer or high-grade precancers. This type of vaccine is designed to boost the immune system so these women can better fight the virus and hence control their disease. This type of vaccine does not rely on antibodies as described above but on a different part of the immune system that uses other cells to fight disease. The second approach is the traditional preventive or prophylactic vaccine that will, we hope, either prevent an individual from becoming infected with HPV in the first place or lessen the impact of a new HPV infection so that HPV precancers or cancers do not develop. These vaccines function by producing infection-fighting antibodies in the person receiving the vaccine. We will discuss each of these approaches in more detail.

Therapeutic or Treatment Vaccines

Therapeutic or treatment vaccines have a different goal than the preventive vaccines created for infectious diseases such as smallpox or hepatitis. Treatment vaccines are designed for use in women who already have severe HPV disease, such as HSIL or cervical cancer. These women have demonstrated that their HPV-caused disease is not going away on its own and that their immune systems are not up to the task of eliminating the virus. It is thought that special therapeutic vaccines may stimulate the woman's immune system to react more strongly to the HPV infection and help precancerous lesions or cancers regress and maybe even go away. These vaccines may also be called "immunotherapy" since they use a woman's own immune system as part of her treatment. It is hoped these therapeutic vaccines could stop the progression of cervical cancer to a fatal stage.

Although the rationale for developing such a treatment vaccine is straightforward, making a successful therapeutic vaccine is a difficult task. Such vaccines are also being pursued for other cancers such as melanoma (a type of skin cancer), for example, but thus far without great success. Cervical cancer is a tumor that can be successfully treated if caught early. Advanced cervical cancer or cancer that isn't cured in the first go-round of treatment can be very difficult to cure with later treatments. There are not a lot of good options for women whose cervical cancer recurs. Immunotherapy may prove to be of value in these women. If it appears effective in cervical cancer patients, there may also be a role for immunotherapy in treating women with HSILs that seem resistant to standard therapy.

To stimulate an immune system for therapeutic vaccine, proteins are used that were made by the virus during the course of infection. These proteins appear to stimulate a different part of a woman's immune system, one that doesn't make antibodies but does make other immune system cells that may fight cancer. No HPV genetic material is included in this vaccine that could cause HPV disease by itself.

There have been several studies looking at the usefulness of therapeutic vaccines in human subjects, in the United States at the National Cancer Institute, in Australia, and in Europe. So far, the results have been mixed but have shown a benefit to at least some patients. Clinical trials have shown at least a few cervical cancer patients whose cancers remained stable with the vaccine or have even regressed. Clinical trials mean that a vaccine has been made and it is currently being tested in human subjects to look at how well it works and the presence of any problematic side effects. Cures of cervical cancer have not been seen. While not a raging success, these clinical trials have been encouraging enough to prompt continued research into immunotherapy. There is some thought that it may be of more benefit in women with less advanced disease, such as women with HSIL. Undoubtedly, we will see more news of therapeutic vaccines for cervical cancer in the future.

Preventive or Prophylactic HPV Vaccines

Considerable progress has been made in the development of a prophylactic HPV vaccine. Monovalent vaccines against HPV 11 and a different one against HPV 16 are both in early clinical trials in the United States and Europe. Development of polyvalent vaccines should take place after mono-valent vaccines are shown to be successful. The current clinical trials are small in scale, involving fewer than two hundred men and women. Study par-ticipants are closely monitored for any side effects from the vaccine. In deter-mining if a vaccine works in these trials, men and women are tested to see if the vaccines produce antibodies traceable to the vaccine. These are anti-bodies that could either prevent them from being infected by HPV or perhaps lead to only a very mild HPV infection that does not produce HPV disease, such as visible genital warts or cervical dysplasia.

If the results from these trials continue to appear favorable in terms of safety and effectiveness, the vaccines will be tried on larger groups. It is only after extensive testing at several different levels that the vaccine trial results are sent to the Federal Drug Administration (FDA) for their review and approval. Not infrequently, the FDA will request additional information or studies. The FDA approval process can be quite lengthy. Only after the FDA is completely satisfied with the vaccine's safety and effectiveness will it be approved for the general public.

The design of these vaccines uses recombinant DNA technology to pro-duce the vaccine, which contains a portion of the outer covering or shell of the virus itself. This is in contrast to the therapeutic vaccine discussed above which used viral proteins from inside the virus. Very important in this vac-cine design is the omission of any intact portion of the virus that could poten-tially reproduce and cause an HPV infection. There is no HPV genetic mate-rial contained within these vaccines. The presence of this HPV outer shell stimulates a person's immune system to produce specific antibodies to the outer covering which, it is hoped, will prevent HPV infection when they are exposed to the virus.

Since HPV 11 is the cause of usually innocuous genital warts with very little likelihood of progressing to cancer, you may wonder why time and money is being spent on an HPV 11 vaccine. Genital warts are actually a major healthcare problem with over 4 million cases a year seen in this country with many of these lesions being resistant to therapy and having a high rate of recurrence. We have already discussed the new pharmacologic or drug approaches to genital warts at the beginning of this chapter.

HPV 11 lesions are also considered "early" HPV lesions and the visible genital wart lesions tend to show up more quickly than precancerous or cancerous lesions caused by high-risk HPV 16 or 18. As has been mentioned, high-grade HPV 16 and 18 lesions may take many years to develop and may be difficult to detect. For these reasons, it should be easier to monitor a vaccine against HPV 11 for efficacy since these lesions develop at a speedier pace.

The results from these vaccine trials are just beginning to be published in the medical literature. The vaccine is being tried on college-aged men and women on university campuses in several different locations across the country. Recently published results from the National Cancer Institute demonstrated that men and women who were vaccinated with an HPV 16 vaccine had HPV 16 antibody levels forty times that seen in naturally infected people. These early trials have brought up several important issues regarding how these vaccines might be used in the future, provided they prove to be successful in safely preventing HPV infection.

First of all, who should receive an HPV vaccine? This question really has two parts: First, at what age should people be immunized against HPV, and second, what sexes should receive the vaccine? As far as the sex issue is concerned, arguments can be made for immunizing both males and females. Such an approach could really strike a decisive blow against the incredibly high incidence of HPV in sexually active individuals. Theoretically, a whole generation of young men and women could be made immune to certain HPV infections. At the moment, however, most vaccine trials are geared to immunizing only women, although men have been included in some studies.

With the issue of age it is clear that people need to be immunized before the start of sexual activity. The most logical age group to start with is preadolescent females. Arguments are also being made for including an HPV vaccine in the regular series of vaccines given to infants and young children. This certainly would be the easiest time to administer the vaccine. Furthermore, in developing countries where a vaccine is needed most, the only opportunity to administer the vaccine may be in this early age group.

The thought of immunizing preadolescent children or even babies against a sexually transmitted disease is bound to raise the hackles of many a parent who is very far from thinking of their children as sexual beings. The ongoing vaccine trials utilizing college-aged women have even run into this major societal issue. However, there is no doubt that immunizing against HPVs early, before boys and girls have had a chance to contract the viruses, is absolutely critical to the vaccine's success.

While the medical researchers charged with developing an effective HPV vaccine have much hard work ahead of them, it is clear that equally hard work will be involved in educating and informing the general public about the need for this medical advance. Parents, particularly parents of girls, will have to look to their children's futures and understand the far-reaching implications and health consequences of HPV infection. They need to understand the widespread prevalence of this infection and learn that their children will most certainly become infected by HPV when they develop into sexually active young adults. Parents need to be informed of the unpredictability of their children's response to an HPV infection. Parents will then have to realize that there is no way of predicting if their children's HPV infection will be a mere passing infection with no ill consequences (other than the continued spread of this cancer-causing virus). Conversely, an HPV infection may result in years of abnormal Pap smears and surgical treatments with all of their emotional and physical side effects or even cause an early, untimely death from cervical cancer.

Informing parents and the general public about HPV is a monumental task for the medical community. Even women with abnormal Pap smears tend to be grossly underinformed about the sexually transmitted nature of the disease for which they are being treated. Most of the women with abnormal Pap smears whom we interviewed for this book had never heard of HPV. The reasons for this lack of information are likely complex but undoubtedly have some basis in the discomfort that discussions of a sexual nature engender on the part of both patients and their physicians. As a society we need to move past the issue of embarrassment about sexual issues and on to the much more important issue of improving the health of our young women and men.

We have spent the last eleven chapters explaining abnormal Pap smears, HPV, and cervical cancer. In the next chapter it is your turn. We focus on specific questions that have come up on these topics during the course of our conversations with women. Hopefully we have included questions that you may have about your particular situation with regard to abnormal Pap smears.

T W E L V E

Your Turn

FREQUENTLY ASKED QUESTIONS ABOUT PAP SMEARS

In the course of researching and writing this book, we quickly learned that even women with previously abnormal Pap smears are frequently not aware of the association between HPV infection and cervical cancer. In an informal survey we conducted of women visiting their gynecologists' offices for Pap smears, we discovered that a majority of women (93 percent) knew that a Pap smear checks for the presence of cervical cancer and most women (59 percent) knew that HPV is a sexually transmitted infection. However, less than a third (32 percent) knew that HPV causes cervical cancer.

Many women we spoke with said that they were never told of the connection between HPV and cervical cancer, even women who had multiple abnormal Pap smears and many procedures for those abnormal results. In fact, some women were not even aware that they had had an HPV infection. When we asked women why they did not ask their clinicians for more information, we were often told that *they did not know what questions to ask.*

In this chapter, we present frequently asked questions about abnormal Pap smears. These questions have been taken from informal chats with women as well as from formal interviews. In addition, we have included questions from women asked during the course of administering our survey. We have also included questions that we would have wanted answered if we were reading a book on abnormal Pap smears.

Our goal here is to answer your questions about abnormal Pap smears, human papillomavirus, cervical precancers, and cervical cancer. We have arranged these questions into topical sections for easy reference. We hope that these will be many of the same questions you may have and that they will prompt you to think of other questions you may want to ask your physician or healthcare provider.

As we stated in the beginning of this book, we firmly believe that you cannot expect to receive optimal health care without being an active and interested participant in that process. Accurate information and open communication with your clinician are the tools that will allow you to discuss your cervical diagnoses intelligently and enable you to be an informed partner in your own health care. As we have seen in our stories of women with cervical disease, it is this type of partnership between you and your clinician that leads to the best and most satisfying medical outcomes.

QUESTIONS ABOUT
HUMAN PAPILLOMAVIRUS INFECTION

Many of the details about HPV infections are confusing, and in our conversations with women certain of their questions about HPV infections keep cropping up time and again. Below are some frequently asked questions about HPV.

Now that my SIL has been treated, am I cured of HPV?

This question brings up some of the puzzling aspects of HPV infection and points out how much of our knowledge about this virus is still in its infancy. HPV researchers postulate several different "levels" of infection although the distinction between these levels can be a bit blurry. Keep in mind that the association between HPV and cervical disease is a relatively recent discovery and researchers have not yet had enough time to understand fully how HPV infections behave over time. An *active clinical HPV infection* indicates that a woman is both infected by HPV *and* has cervical disease as detected by a Pap smear or other means of tissue diagnosis such as a cervical biopsy. There is also *subclinical HPV infection.* By this it is usually meant that although you have an HPV test showing infection by HPV, there is no indication that you have a precancer of the cervix—that is, your Pap smears are normal and no SILs can be found by colposcopy and cervical biopsy. This may be related to a *latent HPV infection* in which HPV is thought to be present in the cervix for an unknown period of time before making its presence known with an abnormal Pap smear or HPV test. Details of HPV latency are still rather sketchy. As for being "cured" of HPV, the majority of women adequately treated for their SILs (active clinical infections) will rid themselves of the virus. SIL treatments themselves, such as laser, cryotherapy, or surgery, seem to invigorate the body's immune system to rid itself of the virus. Most doctors, however, are reluctant to say that women have been "cured" of their HPV infections, since low levels of the virus may still be present, and current technologies may not be able to detect these small amounts of virus. However, most women will have normal HPV tests after successful treatment of their SILs. For all practical purposes, they have probably rid themselves of their infection.

I have been treated for a SIL and all of my Pap smears have since been negative. Is it possible for me to be infected by HPV again or am I now immune?

You certainly can be infected again by HPV. Unlike some other infections, there is no lifelong immunity to HPV that occurs by virtue of once having been infected by the virus. This is because of the different subtypes of genital HPV (more than forty in all), each of which may produce its own special immune response. An immune response to one subtype does not necessarily protect a person from infection by the other subtypes so that you can be reinfected by another HPV subtype. In addition, men and women can be infected by multiple HPV subtypes at one time. You are, however, unlikely to become infected again by the same partner who gave you HPV in the first place. You have most likely mounted an immune response to the subtype or subtypes he infected you with. This immune response will fight off reinfection by that same viral subtype, but you may still be susceptible to infection by other viral subtypes either in different partners or if your same partner becomes infected with other viral subtypes. The fact that there are so many subtypes of genital HPV is somewhat overwhelming. Most of them, however, are fairly rare or found elsewhere in the world, with a smaller subset of subtypes being most common in this country (HPV 6, 11, 16, 18, for example). Your chances of being reexposed to the same HPV subtype (acquired from different men) are actually fairly good and immunity gained from your first exposure will protect you from infection with subsequent exposures. The future success of

HPV vaccines is based on this persistent immunity after exposure to certain HPV subtypes (see chapter 11).

I have a SIL. I have been dealing with this for several years with abnormal Pap smears, cervical biopsies, and loops. I just don't seem to be able to get rid of the SIL. It keeps on coming back. I now have a new boyfriend and am wondering if I can pass it on to him. Is this possible? Should I tell him about my cervical problems?

Since SILs are caused by the sexually transmitted virus HPV, you certainly could pass this virus on to any male with whom you have sex while you are infected. This may not be an issue while the two of you are monogamous but your boyfriend should know that he has been exposed to a very common sexually transmitted virus that he could, in turn, pass on to other women. They could then also be plagued with abnormal Pap smears as you have. Your partner should be aware that this is a silent infection and only rarely causes any symptoms in women and almost never in men. He should be informed that HPV is a virus that can cause cervical cancer in women and can very rarely cause penile cancer in men. We also think you should tell him about this part of your medical history because it so clearly distresses you. In our talks with women, we have found that those with the most social support from friends and family tend to be able to handle their situations with the least amount of anxiety.

Since a SIL reflects a sexually transmitted infection with human papillomavirus, why isn't this infection reported to public health authorities like other sexually transmitted infections such as gonorrhea and chlamydia? Shouldn't infected people contact all their sexual partners and let them know they have been exposed to the virus?

Human papillomavirus is such a common virus in our population of sexually active adults that it would be pointless to list it as a reportable disease to local public-health offices, with a lifetime risk of infection of around 80 percent, according to Dr. Christopher Crum of Harvard Medical School. A key reason that other sexually transmitted diseases are reported to a public health authority is that there exists effective treatment for those infections, generally in the form of antibiotics. As we have discussed, most HPV infections do not need to be treated because a woman's (and presumably a man's) immune system will clear the virus on its own. It is only in a small percent of women (less than 5 percent) that HPV infection causes cervical disease that needs to be treated. These women are identified by virtue of their abnormal Pap smear findings, not because they have been notified about sexual contact with an infected partner. On the contrary, it is women who are usually in the position to inform their male partners that they are infected by HPV. Certainly it is helpful for women to know about being exposed to HPV. We feel that responsible males should inform their female partners if they know they carry HPV, particularly high-risk types, from their previous female partners who have had SILs. If given this information, then a woman should assume she is at risk for cervical precancers and make sure she never misses an annual Pap smear.

Can condoms prevent the spread of HPV? If safe sex works for other sexually transmitted infections, why not HPV?

Actually, this is a common misconception. In our own surveys, nearly 60 percent of women thought that condoms prevented the spread of HPV. Unfortunately, this does not seem to be the case. While condoms covering the penis probably do reduce the spread of HPV, men can carry the virus in areas of their genitals other than just on their penis. For example, the virus may also be present on a man's scrotum, the skin covering his testicles, which is not covered by a condom. Because of this, it is actually possible for a woman to contract HPV from a man by intimate genital contact without actually having sexual intercourse. Vaginal condoms also do not offer protection against HPV for the same reason: they still allow contact with male genital skin. Although not helpful in preventing the spread of HPV, we strongly recommend the practice of safe sex with condoms as is it critical in preventing other serious sexually transmitted infections such as human immunodeficiency virus (HIV), gonorrhea, syphilis, and chlamydia.

I recently was diagnosed with LSIL on my Pap smear and at the same time was told I have chlamydia. Was this determined from my Pap smear? Can these two events be related?

At the same time your Pap smear was taken, your clinician also collected material from your cervix for a chlamydia test, usually done by swabbing your cervix. Chlamydia is a sexually transmitted bacterium that infects the female reproductive organs and if not treated with antibiotics can lead to permanent scarring of those organs and even infertility. Chlamydia infections are detected by a different test than the Pap test, one performed in another part of the medical laboratory, the microbiology lab. Scientists have previously investigated links between chlamydia infection and cervical cancer. Researchers in Finland reported in the *Journal of the American Medical Association* in 2001 that infection by certain types of chlamydia may put women at greater risk for cervical cancer. Other scientists feel this association may not be real because it may be based more on women being sexually active and infected by HPV than by their chlamydia infection.

Can HPV be spread by oral sex?

HPV does not appear to be commonly transmitted through oral sex. This is for the very simple reason that the genital HPVs have an affinity for the human genitals and not other body sites. The exact reasons for this preference are unclear. Medical experts in sexually transmitted diseases, however, do report the very rare occurrence of mouth warts (condylomas) due to genital HPV presumably as a consequence of oral sex. As discussed in a review from England, this rare finding has been noted in the setting of HIV infection and the acquired immunodeficiency infection syndrome (AIDS). For the vast majority of people with healthy immune systems, HPV is not commonly spread by oral sex. HPV can be spread, however, by anal sex. This is discussed in greater depth later in this chapter.

I understand that cervical cancers and precancers are related to infection by human papillomavirus, the wart virus. What is the connection between HPV cervical disease and the warts I frequently get on my hands? I know those warts are also caused by wart viruses. Can I spread the virus from my hands to my cervix? Can I give myself cervical cancer?

You are certainly correct that skin warts, cervical precancers, and cancers are all related to infections by the wart virus, human papillomavirus. Keep in mind, however, that HPV is really a very large family of viruses: currently over 100 different subtypes have been identified. Each HPV type has an area of the body that it likes to infect. The HPV subtypes that cause skin warts or foot warts are acclimated to the outside of our bodies where it is dry and exposed to the air. They cannot survive and infect in areas inside our bodies, areas that provide a very different type of environment, one that is more moist. So, your hand warts cannot spread to your cervix, and a genital HPV type cannot spread to other external parts of your body.

I have been treated for a SIL over the past few years and have also been unsuccessful in becoming pregnant. Could my infertility be related to my SIL and infection by HPV?

HPV infections and SILs themselves are not known to be associated with infertility in either men or women. There are complications of treatment of SILs, however, which can on rare occasions lead to problems conceiving and in maintaining a pregnancy once a woman has conceived. Surgical procedures such as cervical cones, loops, laser therapy, and cryotherapy can all lead to cervical narrowing (stenosis). Rarely with this condition, the cervix becomes so scarred and narrowed that sperm may have difficulty traveling up into a woman's uterus and fallopian tubes where conception occurs. This complication can be successfully treated with special instruments to dilate the cervix. Another complication, seen more often with extensive cervical surgery such as cervical cones, is cervical incompetence. This condition can result in a cervix that has difficulty staying closed when a woman is pregnant, thereby leading to problems with miscarriages, though this condition is uncommon. An incompetent cervix can be treated after a woman is pregnant by tight stitching of the cervix so that it will stay closed and a pregnancy remains in place.

I am forty years old, single, and want to have a child. I am planning to use a sperm bank to conceive. Is there any risk of contracting HPV from a sperm donor?

A recent study from Canada points out that current guidelines for screening potential sperm donors do not include HPV testing. Through this study it was noted that HPV was present in sperm from donors with no outward signs of infection and that the virus was still present after the conventional "sperm washing" performed by donor insemination programs. This suggests that there is a risk of HPV transmission to women from donated infected sperm, however, there have been no documented cases of HPV lesions resulting from HPV transmission to a donor-sperm recipient. It may be a good idea to ask for HPV testing of any donated sperm.

Is genital HPV infection similar to genital herpes where the virus can be passed to an infant during the birthing process?

Fortunately, there is not the same concern about transmission of HPV during delivery of a baby as there is with genital herpes. Millions of women infected (most unknowingly) with HPV give birth to healthy babies. Of course, in medicine we can always find exceptions. There is a very rare condition known as *juvenile laryngeal papilloma*, in which children are noted to have warty growths in their throats. Genital HPV subtypes are present in these warts and it is thought that they are due to the rare passage of HPV from an infected mother to her infant during delivery. Thankfully, this is a very rare event and, unlike herpes, there are no precautions necessary during labor and delivery for a woman with HPV.

What about gay men and HPV? Do they have any problems with this infection?

You are quite right in that a distinction should be made between heterosexual and homosexual men when discussing the effects of genital HPV. As mentioned previously, heterosexual men can be infected with HPV; however, they experience very few consequences of this infection, as compared to women. Very, very rarely HPV lesions on the penis can lead to penis cancer. This relative freedom from the ill effects of HPV is not true for homosexual men. With differing sexual practices, such as anal sex, gay men commonly experience HPV infection of the skin around the anus. This area actually has similarities to a woman's cervical transformation zone, the area preferred by HPV and where cervical dysplasia arises. In one study from the University of California, San Francisco, a large number of gay men (around 60 percent) carry HPV in this area (often several HPV subtypes at once) and the number jumps up to well over 90 percent in gay men who are infected by HIV. In recent years, medical personnel have noted a startling increase in anal cancer in gay men with about double the rate of anal cancer in gay men with HIV compared to those without HIV. It is thought that, as with cervical cancer, HPV infection in the anal area is a factor in the development of anal cancer.

To put the numbers of anal cancer cases in perspective, the scientists at the University of California, San Francisco, suggest that gay men are getting HPV-related anal cancer at a rate close to that of cervical cancer prior to the introduction of the Pap smear. We are starting to see in our practices "anal Pap smears" taken from gay men as a screening test for anal precancers. Women who engage in anal intercourse, particularly women with vulvar, vaginal, or cervical SILs or who are infected with HIV, may also be at risk for anal cancer.

AGE, REPRODUCTIVE STATUS, AND ABNORMAL PAP SMEARS

Women of any age can have atypical Pap smears. In this section we address questions that may arise in women of varying ages who have received atypical Pap smears.

My daughter is fifteen years old and has been dating for about six months. I gather some of her friends are having sex with their boyfriends and I am concerned my daughter may soon do the same. We have discussed both abstinence and birth control. Does she need a Pap smear?

Your daughter is fortunate to have a mother who is openly communicating with her about her developing sexuality. Certainly unwanted pregnancy is a big concern and birth control should be available for male and female teens who are sexually active. Your daughter also needs to hear about the sexually transmitted infections that are increasingly prevalent in the teen population. Sexually transmitted bacterial infections, such as gonorrhea, syphilis, and chlamydia are surprisingly widespread in some communities, crossing all socioeconomic lines. These infections may have some characteristic symptoms such as a vaginal discharge or sores. Some infections, however, such as chlamydia in particular, may not have any symptoms and can silently spread up her cervix to infect her uterus, her fallopian tubes, and her ovaries, which may result in infertility later on in life. Your daughter also needs to know about sexually transmitted viral infections such as herpes simplex virus and human papillomavirus. Once acquired, both of these can infect a female for life (herpes) or for several months to years (HPV). Herpes results in a symptomatic infection with painful genital sores, but HPV is most often a silent infection with no symptoms. HPV is certainly the more common of the two and unlike herpes, it is a virus with the potential to cause cervical cancer. Infection by HPV in teens is more likely to result in cervical precancers than in older women with the same infection. If infected by HPV, she will not only have an infection that she could pass on to other sexual partners but an infection that could lead to cervical precancers and then to cancer. Once any female becomes sexually active, it is time to sign up for regular Pap smears. While suggesting abstinence may be an unpopular idea, we applaud any parent for taking this brave position. Young teenage girls need to hear about abstinence as an alternative to risky sexual practices that can potentially lead to infertility and even cancer. There will be time enough for sexual experimentation when girls attain both emotional and cervical maturity! We must continue to emphasize, however, that women of any age are susceptible to the effects of HPV.

I am about five months pregnant and concerned about my Pap smear taken early in my pregnancy. The diagnosis was "atypical cells of undetermined significance, favor low-grade squamous intraepithelial lesion." I had a similar Pap smear diagnosis about a year ago but I became pregnant before I did anything about it. Will being pregnant have any effect on this?

With two identical atypical Pap smear diagnoses waving red flags about the possibility of a SIL, you should be concerned that you may have an HPV infection, which resulted in precancerous changes in your cervix. Unfortunately, pregnancy is not an ideal time to investigate this possibility in any complete way. Your gynecologist can perform colposcopy to inspect your cervix visually and may even perform cervical biopsies. Examination of your endocervical canal, however, is generally not undertaken because your canal must stay closed to protect your pregnancy. This leaves the possibility of an undetected SIL higher up in your canal. Even if the above steps confirm a SIL, your doctor will most likely wait until after you deliver your baby to evaluate you completely. It is difficult to predict if pregnancy will have any effect on this problem. This depends on if the SIL is sensitive to pregnancy hormones. Some women experience complete regression of their HPV lesions during pregnancy while other women see persistence and even progression to more severe lesions.

I just had my second child. At my check-up, six weeks after my delivery, I had a Pap smear that came back "atypical." What is going on? I have always had normal Pap smears and have had the same sexual partner for eight years.

Pregnancy is a time of marked hormonal changes in women and it may take awhile before your body returns to its normal nonpregnant hormonal state. These changes can be reflected in atypical changes in your cervix. We have also seen these atypical cells in women who have recently aborted or miscarried. These changes can look quite worrisome and may resemble SILs. In the vast majority of women these atypical changes resolve over a few months as their bodies return to their normal hormonal state. In any event, women with pregnancy-related atypical results should return for a repeat Pap smear in three to six months. By that time atypical results due to postpartum hormonal effects will have resolved, but if the results were due to HPV it should persist. A woman with a second abnormal Pap smear would then be a candidate for more in-depth follow-up with cervical colposcopy and biopsies.

I am a forty-five-year-old woman who has always had normal Pap smears. Several years ago, I started getting atypical Pap smears. Nothing has changed in my life, other than getting older! I have the same partner I have had for the past eighteen years. What is going on?

You are giving a perfect description of what can happen to a woman's Pap smears as she approaches menopause. This phase of a woman's life is called "perimenopause" and although you may still be having periods, your body is experiencing changes in levels of your sex hormones—estrogen and progesterone. The lining of your cervix is also susceptible to changes in your hormone levels and the cells there can undergo changes that mimic SILs. Due to these hormonal changes, women at this time of life may end up with abnormal Pap smears with no underlying cervical disease. At the same time, however, older women with atypical Pap smears are worrisome because if these abnormalities reflect the presence of HPV, these infections may have persisted for many years, evading the ability of the woman's immune system to eliminate them. It is in this setting that cervical cancer can result. Perimenopausal women with repeated atypical Pap smears may be ideal candidates for HPV testing to resolve this confusing situation.

I am a postmenopausal woman. I have not had a period in fifteen years and am not on hormone replacement therapy. I am not sexually active. I was just told my Pap smear is abnormal. Do I need to worry about this?

One common cause of atypical Pap smears in older women is "post-menopausal atypia." Due to the changes in levels of hormones during menopause, the Pap smear of an older woman may show the effects of low estrogen levels on her cervix. Low estrogen produces a Pap smear that can have some of the features we look for in cervical precancers—enlarged and darker nuclei that take up more of the cell. We call these changes "atrophy," and they look very different compared to the cells of a woman who is of reproductive age with lots of estrogen. Sometimes these atrophic changes can result in enlarged nuclei with irregular shapes, which bring to mind cervical precancers. While we can usually be fairly sure these changes are all due to a woman being postmenopausal, they may be present to such an extent that we are concerned about a SIL. Due to the similarities in cell changes in atrophy and precancer, it can be difficult to detect a true cervical SIL in a background of atrophy. It is at this point that we will diagnose a Pap smear as being atypical with a recommendation for a repeat Pap smear. In such situations, we will also often request that the woman undergo an "estrogen test," a short course of vaginal estrogen cream. Application of the cream into the vagina over several weeks will act to change an atrophic cervix back to one resembling a younger woman where a SIL is easier to detect. The Pap smear should be repeated immediately (within several days) after the vaginal cream is stopped. Within a few days of stopping the cream, a postmenopausal woman's cervix will start to look atrophic again with the same problems in detecting a SIL. Actually, older women with these changes are ideal candidates for HPV testing. If an older woman tests positive for HPV, it most likely means she has had a persistent infection for a number of years and is therefore at high risk for cervical cancer. Since HPV can persist for years after the initial infection, you do not need to currently be sexually active to have precancerous or cancerous changes in your cervix as a result of HPV.

I am in my late fifties have recently started taking hormonal replacements. For the first time in my life I recently had an atypical Pap smear. Could the hormonal replacement therapy be causing my atypical Pap smears?

Hormone replacement therapy in postmenopausal women is not known to result in atypical Pap smears. Regardless of the hormone replacement therapy, you are still a postmenopausal woman and can be susceptible to the same postmenopausal atypia that we described in the question above. Sometimes hormone replacement therapy will result in a very "young" looking Pap smear in that the extra estrogen will cause your cervical cells to look like cells from a reproductive-age woman. Other times a Pap smear from a woman on hormone replacement will still look atrophic and perhaps contain atypical cells. Whatever your Pap smear looks like, you still need to follow-up an atypical Pap smear with a repeat smear in three to six months.

I had my uterus removed five years ago. My doctor still wants me to come in to have a Pap smear every year. Is this really necessary since I don't have a uterus anymore?

You bring up several important issues. First, we know that a woman's annual visit to her doctor for her Pap smear and pelvic examination is often the only time women will see a physician. It is at these visits that you are examined for many other things in addition to being screened for cervical cancer by having your Pap smear. Your physician may check your general health with blood pressure and weight measurements and by listening to your heart. She will probably examine your breasts for breast cancer as well as ask you about other areas of your health. A physician may also perform a quick urine test to check for illnesses such as diabetes and kidney disease. They will also perform a pelvic examination in order to conduct a Pap smear but also to make sure your ovaries are normal in size and to assess your outer genitals. Second, although you had your uterus removed by a hysterectomy, you need to know if your cervix and ovaries were removed at the same time. Ovaries are not always removed at the time of hysterectomy, particularly in younger women who may have a number of years remaining of good ovarian function. The ovaries can still secrete sex hormones even if the uterus has been removed. If your ovaries were not removed, you still need a pelvic examination to make sure they are normal size. Although rarely done today, in the past hysterectomies for benign problems (such as a "dropping" uterus, also known as uterine prolapse) sometimes left a woman's cervix behind in what is called a "supracervical" hysterectomy. If your cervix is still present, your doctor has been performing regular cervical Pap smears and you should continue to have these annually. If it is surgically removed, your doctor has been scraping the wall of your vagina for your Pap smear. Vaginal Pap smears are done in women with hysterectomies to screen for the possibility of vaginal squamous cell cancer or precancers. Recall that HPV can infect vaginal tissue and also lead to cancer in that site. There is some controversy about the need for older women with hysterectomies to continue having vaginal Pap smears if they have never had atypical Pap smears in the past. One study by the Louisiana State University Medical Center showed very little value in continuing Pap smears in this older age group. A very small number of women in this study were found to have vaginal precancers or cancers. This is a situation where a single HPV test may be very valuable in determining the need to continue Pap tests. Sexually active younger women with hysterectomies should be considered still at risk for HPV infection, which may lead to vaginal and vulvar precancers, and they should continue their vaginal Pap smears.

I am a gay woman and have never had sex with a man. Do I need a Pap smear?

HPV infection is most commonly transmitted through sex between a man and a woman. While you may not have ever had sex with a man, the same may not be true for your female partner(s). Studies from the University of California, Los Angeles, and Duke University have shown that over 70 percent of lesbians have previously had male sexual partners. All it takes is one male partner to acquire HPV. According to a physician who cares for gay women, there are some positions that gay women may engage in during sex that could possibly transmit HPV from one woman to another if one woman is infected. HPV is known to be able to be spread on sex toys as well. Having said all this, gay women are generally considered to be at lower risk than heterosexual women for HPV infection, precancers, and cancer. To be considered low risk, however, a gay woman (or a straight woman for that matter) should fulfill certain criteria: no more than five male sexual partners during her lifetime, no previous atypical Pap smears of a severity that required colposcopy (such as a SIL or multiple ASCUSs), and no previous sexually transmitted infections. If these criteria are met, some physicians feel that a woman can go to a two- to three-year schedule for Pap smears. Other physicians, however, feel that an annual Pap smear is still the safest route. Talk to your healthcare provider about your risks and how often he or she recommends you have a Pap smear performed.

RISK FACTORS FOR CERVICAL CANCER

In several places in this book we have touched on the various risk factors for cervical cancer. The following questions will serve to emphasize the importance of evaluating your own personal risk factors for this disease.

I am sixteen and my boyfriend and I are holding off having sex. We do go in for some pretty heavy petting but we haven't had sex. Do I still need a Pap smear?

With deference to Bill Clinton, HPV does not need "real" sex with full vaginal penetration and ejaculation to be transmitted between two individuals. In addition to carrying the virus in the cells lining their penis, men may carry HPV in the outer skin of their penis and scrotum and the rest of their genital skin. They can pass the virus to women simply by the physical contact of their genitals. This is why condoms do not stop the spread of HPV. If your boyfriend has had other sexual contacts he may well carry the virus and could pass it to you even without vaginal penetration. In addition to acquiring cervical SILs from HPV, women can less commonly acquire HPV precancers in their vulva and vagina. As in the cervix, if due to high-risk HPV types such infections also run a risk of progression to invasive cancer if left untreated. Unfortunately, the vulva and vagina are not tested during a routine Pap smear and an HPV infection in those sites may go undetected. This is because it would not be possible to scrape the entire surface of the vagina and vulva. Keep in mind that cancer occurs much less frequently in these sites. A trained gynecologist can recognize possible abnormalities in the vagina and vulva during a visual genital examination performed at the same time as a Pap smear. If an abnormality is sighted, a biopsy can be taken from that area. It is not too early to start regular gynecologic examinations, which include a genital examination and Pap smear.

I am a cigarette smoker and have always had normal Pap smears. Why does my gynecologist put "cigarette smoking" on my Pap smear form as a "risk factor"?

This is because laboratories encourage doctors to tell us which of their patients are at higher risk for cervical cancer. As a smoker, you are in a higher risk category for developing cervical cancer. Compounds present in cigarette smoke such as nitrosamines seem to have the ability to affect cervical cells infected by HPV and could cause them to more easily develop precancerous and cancerous changes. Other factors that place women into "higher risk" categories for cervical cancer include having sexual intercourse at an early age (prior to age fifteen), having a number of sexual partners (at any age), having had abnormal Pap smears in the past, having other sexually trans-mitted diseases, and being on oral contraceptives.

I have not had a sexual partner in over three years. I also don't have any health insurance and my last physical examination was about five years ago. Since I am not sexually active, do I need a Pap smear? I am in very good health and don't feel the need for checkups.

While you may now be the picture of health, you still could have a persistent HPV infection lurking in your genital tract. Just recall the high prevalence of HPV infection with 25 to 45 percent of sexually active women infected. Keep in mind that most of the cases of cervical cancer in our country are found in women who haven't had a Pap smear in the past three to five years. Their SILs had that period of time to go undetected and progress unchecked. It is unfortunate that it is often the women at risk and who most need Pap smears who are least able to afford them. Most cities or counties have either state or municipal public health services that offer pelvic examinations and Pap smears at a very reduced cost or free of charge provided to women without health insurance or with limited financial resources. Find the clinic nearest you and make an appointment for a test. At the same time make sure that you have a full pelvic examination that checks the size of your ovaries and uterus and have a breast examination.

I am concerned because my mother died five years ago from cervical cancer and both my sisters have HSILs. Can cervical cancer run in my family?

This is an excellent question. Although not nearly as well defined as the familial link in other cancers, such as some breast and colon cancers, there are some indications that certain families may be at higher risk for cervical cancer. Some of the current research in cervical cancer, such as that con-ducted at the University of New Mexico and in Sweden, is investigating genetic links in the disease. Some of this is focusing on the particulars of women's immune systems and their susceptibilities to cervical cancer. Such features of the immune system are ones that you inherit from your parents. We can safely say that your mother and your sisters all had persistent HPV infections that their immune systems were not able to completely clear. Although your immune system may be completely capable of successfully fighting HPV, through your blood relationships, you share some of the same immune system components with other females in your family. We are still unclear about this connection but you probably should consider yourself at risk for cervical cancer and never miss a Pap smear. You might want to have yourself tested for HPV to ensure you do not have a persistent infection. You haven't mentioned other aspects of your life important in assessing cervical cancer risk (smoking, number of sexual partners, age at first intercourse) but all of those figure into a complete assessment of your risk.

I am forty-five years old and am a DES daughter. I know I am at greater risk for cervical cancer. Does this mean that DES makes me more susceptible to HPV infection?

You are absolutely correct in that you are at greater risk for cervical cancer by being a DES (diethylstilbestrol) daughter. This was a drug that many pregnant women took in the 1950s to prevent miscarriage. It has long been discontinued since it was realized that the daughters of women who took the drug (and hence were exposed to the drug in utero) were at higher risk for vaginal and cervical cancer. The types of vaginal and cervical cancer that DES daughters tend to get are different from the HPV-related cancers that occur in those sites. Rather than squamous cell carcinoma, DES daughters can get a very rare sort of cervical and vaginal cancer called "clear-cell carcinoma," actually a type of adenocarcinoma (a cancer of glandular tissue). The good news is that only a very small number of DES daughters (less than 0.1 percent) develop adenocarcinoma. Most of them develop it at a young age, between the ages of fifteen and twenty. You, at age forty-five are probably out of the danger zone; however, women who are DES daughters need their regular cervical Pap smears, and it might also be wise to follow them with vaginal smears. These latter smears look for atypical glandular cells in the vagina, a site where typically no glandular tissue exists at all. The process of cancer in DES daughters appears independent of HPV and the risk factors associated with that infection. In essence, if you are a DES daughter, you need to be doubly wise. You could get squamous cell precancers from HPV infection and still be at risk for the rare clear-cell carcinoma through your DES exposure.

UNDERSTANDING YOUR PAP SMEAR DIAGNOSIS

One of the more difficult features of Pap smears is understanding what your diagnosis means. This is particularly true due to the changes that have occurred in Pap smear terminology over the past twenty years. The following questions bring up some issues regarding Pap smear diagnoses and terminology.

I was recently diagnosed with cervical cancer. Fortunately it had not invaded and I have been told I am most likely cured of my cancer after my loop. Can I ever get cervical cancer again?

You bring up two excellent points about Pap smear terminology and HPV infection. First, you have just mentioned a common misunderstanding about cervical precancers and cancer. It is important to realize that in today's terminology a noninvasive cervical cancer is called a high-grade squamous intraepithelial lesion or HSIL. The older terminology called one type of HSIL cervical squamous carcinoma in-situ which may be where you got the impression of a cancer diagnosis. Your lesion is more appropriately considered a cervical precancer than cervical cancer. If we rephrase your question about the possibility of getting SIL again, the answer is a definite yes. There is the chance that your entire original lesion was not completely excised and can grow back. Although a woman may have successful treatment of a SIL, there is also the possibility of being reinfected by a different subtype HPV, particularly from a new partner, and again being diagnosed with a SIL.

I have just been diagnosed with something called AIS. What is this?

AIS stands for adenocarcinoma in-situ which refers to a noninvasive lesion of your endocervical glands. AIS is also due to HPV and is equivalent to a high-grade dysplasia of your endocervix. Recall that your endocervical glands line your cervix high up in the canal leading to your uterus. Although much less common (by more than 75 percent), this tissue is also susceptible to the cancer-causing effect of HPV. It tends to be the same high-risk HPV types that cause high-grade squamous lesions in your cervix that cause problems in your endocervix. In fact, about 50 percent of women with AIS also have a simultaneous HSIL present adjacent in their cervix. The problem with AIS lesions is that while they can be diagnosed on a Pap smear they can be very difficult or near impossible to see by colposcopy. Treatment often requires a full-blown surgical cone to ensure complete removal. Just as with HSIL, AIS has a definite risk of progression to an invasive cancer.

I was recently told I have VIN III. Can this lead to cancer?

VIN lesions or vulvar intraepithelial neoplasia lesions are intimately related to SILs. This lesion is essentially a SIL occurring on your vulva rather than your cervix. Your vulva consists of your external genitalia such as your labia and it is another place that HPV likes to infect. The fact that HPV can reside in a woman's vulva and vagina illustrates how difficult HPV may be to eradicate from a woman's reproductive organs. When a woman has an HPV lesion in her vagina it is called vaginal intraepithelial lesion or VAIN. Just like cervical SILs, both VINs and VAINs are classified as being high- or low-grade. VIN III and VAIN III are high-grade lesions analogous to an HSIL on your cervix. Like an HSIL, a VIN or VAIN can lead to cancer. Just like SILs, VINs and VAINs need to be treated, usually by surgical excision or laser.

I have just received a negative Pap smear. Does that mean that I am free of ovarian as well as cervical cancer? My mother's sister died of ovarian cancer and I am terrified of dying of it, too.

The Pap smear was designed primarily to screen for cervical cancer. Although it is occasionally possible to diagnose an endometrial cancer and, very rarely, an ovarian cancer by Pap smear, this test is not the best way to check for ovarian cancer. If you have a family history of ovarian cancer, you will want to inform your gynecologist of this fact as ovarian cancer can run in families. He or she may want to discuss other studies with you such as periodic ultrasound exams to look at your ovaries. A normal Pap smear does not mean that your ovaries have been given a clean bill of health.

In this chapter we have hopefully touched on the more common questions you may have had about abnormal Pap smears and cervical cancer. If you do not see your question here, ask your physician during your next appointment. Another resource is the medical director of the cytology laboratory that reads your Pap smears. He or she can answer your Pap smear and HPV-related questions. Questions about treatment, however, are best deferred to your clinician.

THIRTEEN

Understanding Your Abnormal Pap Smear

In the first chapter of this book we met Karen, a woman in her early thirties who has just learned that she has an abnormal Pap smear. Like most women, she understands that Pap smears test for cervical cancer and her first response is to panic. However, at her follow-up appointment she learns that she does not in fact have cancer but instead has a *pre*cancerous lesion. *What in the world is a pre-cancer?* Karen doesn't understand this term and finds the explanations confusing. She is told that her actual diagnosis is low-grade SIL and she needs to return for a colposcopy in two weeks. After she leaves her doctor's office, Karen decides to learn as much as she can about her cervical disease and stumbles upon this book.

In chapter 1 she learns that the Pap smear can see changes in cells that are diagnostic for either cervical cancer or cervical cancer precursors called SILs. These changes in the cervix come about because of a sexually transmitted infection by the human papillomavirus or HPV. Karen is astonished to learn that this virus is the most common sexually transmitted infection in the United States and nearly 80 percent of sexually active individuals are thought to have had this infection at one time. She is relieved to learn about the concept of latency in which the virus is thought to be able to remain in a person's body for an unspecified period of time. Karen has not had sex with anyone other than her husband for the past eight years and is relatively confident that her husband has been faithful to her as well. In theory, if she has an HPV infection, she could have contracted it in college, where she had multiple sexual partners before she married her husband.

Although Karen is fairly sure about how she could have developed an

HPV infection, she is less sure about *where* her infection is. In chapter 2 she learns that her cervix is the lower part of her uterus, the passageway into the vagina. She also learns how a Pap smear is taken and how it is interpreted. It seems incredible that hundreds of thousands of her cells end up on a slide for the Pap smear test. In chapter 3 Karen learns about the two cell types that can be seen on a Pap smear and the meaning of Pap smear diagnoses. She decides to ask her doctor's office to send her her own Pap smear report so that she can read the diagnosis for herself.

Karen's report arrives a week later and she sees that the diagnosis is written as:

LOW-GRADE SQUAMOUS INTRAEPITHELIAL LESION
SATISFACTORY FOR EVALUATION BUT
LIMITED BY OBSCURING INFLAMMATION

RECOMMEND REPEAT PAP SMEAR IN 3–6 MONTHS, COL-
POSCOPY OR OTHER FOLLOW-UP AS CLINICALLY INDICATED

From her reading, Karen knows that the changes seen in her Pap smear are diagnostic of an LSIL that is caused by an HPV infection. She understands that this diagnosis is one that can be handled by a repeat Pap smear or by moving on to a closer view of her cervix known as colposcopy with cervical biopsies depending on the opinion of her clinician. Karen's clinician wants to move straight to colposcopy and cervical biopsy. Karen is also somewhat worried about her Pap smear's adequacy which was read as "limited." She now knows that this means that anywhere from 50 to 75 percent of her slide was covered by inflammation and could not be assessed. Could this mean that even worse cellular changes are hiding underneath the inflammation? Is it still possible that she has cervical cancer?

In chapter 4 Karen learns about the various types of treatments that are available for SILs. By reading the stories of women who have undergone colposcopy, she feels she is ready for this procedure that she knows will be painless. She is a little nervous about the biopsies, anticipating that they may cause her some pain. She has already spoken to her doctor's office to ask if she can take some pain reliever before her procedure. She arranges to take the afternoon off from work and is bringing a good friend with her to drive her home and to provide moral support. Her husband will come home early and take care of dinner and the kids' homework.

Karen's colposcopy goes smoothly and her physician takes three biopsies of areas that look "a little funny" as well as an endocervical curettage. Fortunately, Karen experiences very little pain and just a little bleeding. The hard part is waiting for the diagnosis. In just over a week after her procedure, she once again goes to her doctor's office for a follow-up appointment. This time she brings her husband with her to the appointment. Her biopsies in fact show that she has an HSIL, the lesion that is most at-risk for progressing to cancer. She recalls from reading chapter 4 that a minority of women who have LSIL diagnoses on their Pap smears will actually have HSILs on their biopsies because Pap smears only sample very superficial cells. Her endocervical curettage is negative meaning that there is no evidence of HSIL in her endocervical canal. Karen now needs to have a cervical loop procedure.

Karen has read chapter 6, the chapter that deals with cervical cancer. She realizes that an early cancer of the cervix may appear to be just an HSIL on a few biopsies and it is only when the entire cervix is examined that the diagnosis of early cancer can be made. She prays that this is not the case with her but carefully reads the chapter.

Karen's loop procedure is done and she recovers quietly at home. Karen is surprised at how tired she is and how much pain she is in on the first day. After reading some of the women's stories in chapter 7, she decides not to be a martyr and takes the full amount of pain medication prescribed for her. She is better in just a few short days and again grimly begins the hard part: the agony of waiting for her pathology results. She calls a few sympathetic friends who offer her support.

At her physician's office two weeks later, she is shocked to learn that her HSIL was extensive and involved nearly the whole surface of her cervix specimen. Fortunately, the edges or "margins" were clear of HSIL so it looked as if her entire lesion had been removed. Relief washes over her as she leaves her doctor's office. She has a sobering thought: it is clear to her that her HSIL could have quietly progressed into a cancer if she had neglected to have her Pap smear. Although most cervical cancers take years to progress to malignancy, Karen knows this is not always the case. If she had delayed getting a Pap smear for a year or two, her treatment and her life might have followed a very different course. She makes a mental note to quiz her two sisters and her teenaged niece to make sure that *their* Pap smears are up-to-date.

For the time being, Karen is relieved to be finished with this particular chapter in her life. She now encourages all her friends to have their yearly Pap smears without delay and tells them about her experience. After all the reading Karen has done on Pap smears, she is also very knowledgeable about cervical terminology and treatments and readily passes that knowledge on to her friends who have abnormal Pap smears. After her own cervical problems began, Karen discovered that a number of her friends have had abnormal Pap smears at some point in their lives.

Karen also read chapter 10 on lifestyle and cervical cancer prevention. She reflects on her lifestyle and feels relieved that her life has minimal added risks of cervical cancer. She does have friends who smoke cigarettes and decides to inform them of their increased risk of cervical cancer in hopes they may have additional motivation to quit.

As mentioned, Karen is not a real person. However, the many real women who spoke with us about their cervical problems were glad that their stories could help others. They wanted us to share their experiences in this book so that other women could learn from them. All agreed that no woman should be afraid when receiving her abnormal Pap smear diagnosis. We couldn't agree more. We also would encourage you to take charge of your body and learn as much as you can about your diagnosis. We strongly feel that it is important to pass on what you know about cervical disease to other women. We hope that in the very near future, all women will understand their risks of cervical cancer and how to avoid this preventable disease.

A P P E N D I X A

Questions for Your Doctor

I. QUESTIONS ABOUT YOUR PAP SMEAR

1. What was the Pap smear diagnosis?
2. Was the Pap smear satisfactory for the laboratory to examine?
3. If not, what was the reason for it being less than satisfactory?
4. Were endocervical cells present on the Pap smear?
5. Was any specific infection identified?
6. Was inflammation present?
7. Were there any other comments given about the Pap smear?
8. Does the Pap smear need to be repeated?
9. What do you recommend for follow-up of this Pap smear?

II. QUESTIONS ABOUT YOUR COLPOSCOPY AND CERVICAL BIOPSY

1. What did you see during colposcopy?
2. How many biopsies did you take?
3. Was an endocervical curettage performed?
4. What were the results of the biops(y/ies) and curettage?
5. If inflammation was reported on the pathology reports, does this need to be treated?
6. Were any of the specimens considered too scanty for diagnosis?

7. Did any of the biopsy results indicate that the transformation zone was not sampled?
8. Does the biopsy and/or curettage need to be repeated?
9. What do you recommend for follow-up of these results?

III. QUESTIONS ABOUT YOUR LOOP OR CONE

1. What diagnosis was given for this specimen?
2. If SIL was present, was it completely removed? Were the margins free of SIL?
3. What were the results of the endocervical curettage?
4. Were any of the specimens indicated as being too scanty for diagnosis?
5. Was the transformation zone sampled in my loop procedure?
6. Does the procedure need to be repeated?
7. What do you recommend for follow-up?

IV. QUESTIONS ABOUT YOUR CERVICAL CANCER, BEFORE TREATMENT

1. What type of cancer do I have?
2. Is it truly invasive cancer or is it an in-situ lesion?
3. How deeply does the tumor invade?
4. How large is the tumor?
5. Does the tumor show invasion of blood or lymph vessels?
6. Are you trained to treat women with cervical cancer?
7. If not, can you refer me to a gynecologic oncologist?
8. What type of treatment do you recommend?
9. Will surgery be necessary and if so, what type?
10. What will be removed during the surgery? Will lymph nodes be removed?
11. How long will I be in the hospital?
12. How long will it take for me to recover from the surgery? How long will I be out from work?
13. If radiation therapy is planned, will it come before or after surgery?

14. How long will the radiation therapy last?
15. Do I need chemotherapy?
16. What chemotherapy drugs will be used and what are their side effects?
17. How long will I need to take chemotherapy?
18. What are my chances of survival?
19. Can you recommend a support group for women with cancer?

V. QUESTIONS ABOUT YOUR CERVICAL CANCER, AFTER TREATMENT

1. What were the pathology results from my surgery?
2. Was the tumor completely removed?
3. Does the tumor show invasion of blood or lymph vessels?
4. If lymph nodes were removed, did they show metastatic tumor?
5. What additional treatment do I need?
6. How often should I be seen for follow-up of this cancer?
7. What does the follow-up entail? Physical examination, repeat Pap smears from the site of surgery, CT scans?
8. What are my chances of survival now that I have been treated?

Pap Smear Log

Name: _____

Date	Pap Smear Diagnosis	Adequacy	Physician/Clinic	Comments	Follow-up

SAMPLE PAP SMEAR LOG

A P P E N D I X B

Additional Information

GENERAL REFERENCES ON WOMEN'S HEALTH

Boston's Women's Health Book Collective. 1998. *Our Bodies Ourselves for the New Century.* New York: Simon and Schuster.

Carlson, K. J., S. A. Eisenstat, and T. Ziporyn. 1996. *The Harvard Guide to Women's Health.* Cambridge, Mass.: Harvard University Press.

Epps, R. P., and S. C. Stewart, eds. 1995. *American Medical Women's Association: The Women's Complete Health Book.* New York: Dell.

Scialli, A. R., ed. 1999. *The National Women's Health Resource Center Book of Women's Health: Your Comprehensive Guide to Health and Well-Being.* New York: William Morrow and Co.

GENERAL REFERENCES FOR A HEALTHY LIFESTYLE

Brown, E. E. 1973. *Tassajara Cooking.* Boulder, Colo.: Shambhala Publications, Inc.

Kaehler, K., and C. K. Olson. 1999. *Real-World Fitness.* New York: Golden Books.

Madison, D. 1997. *Vegetarian Cooking for Everyone.* New York: Broadway Books.

McGraw, A. 1994. *Yoga, Mind, Body.* Warner Home Video.

Simonds, N. 1999. *A Spoonful of Ginger: Irresistible, Health-giving Recipes from Asian Kitchens.* New York: Alfred A. Knopf.

Tribole, E. 1998. *Stealth Health: How to Sneak Nutrition Painlessly into Your Diet.* New York: Viking Penguin.

Willett, W. 2001. *Eat, Drink, and Be Healthy.* New York: Simon & Schuster.

WEB SITES AND PHONE NUMBERS FOR INFORMATION ABOUT PAP SMEARS, HPV, AND SILs

American College of Obstetricians and Gynecologists: www.acog.org

American Social Health Association (ASHA): www.ashastd.org

ASHA HPV Hotline: 1-877-HPV-5868

ASHA Web site for teens: www.iwannaknow.org

Centers for Disease Control and Prevention, National Breast and Cervical Cancer Early Detection Program: www.cdc.gov/cancer/nbccedp/index.htm

Cervical Dysplasia Support Group: www.egroups.com/group/cervical_dysplasia

E-mail reminders to get a Pap smear: www.papsmear.org

Louisiana State University Medical Center: www.lib-sh.lsumc.edu/fammed/ atlases/ colpo.html

Microsoft Network: www.communities.msn.com/DiagnosisCervicalDysplasia/home

National Cancer Institute Cancer Information Service, Breast and Cervical Cancer Detection and Control Program (for information on sources of low-cost Pap test): 1-800-422-6237

Obstetrics and Gynecology Forum: www.forums.obgyn.net/womens-health/WHF. 9811.html

PlainSense: www.plainsense.com/Health/Womens/papsmear.htm

Planned Parenthood: www.plannedparenthood.org/sti/HPVfacts. html

University of Nebraska: www.unmc.edu/GME/Colp/COba6001.htm

WEB SITES AND PHONE NUMBERS FOR INFORMATION ABOUT CERVICAL CANCER

American Cancer Society: www.cancer.org/; 1-800-227-2345

Cancer Service Information: web.kcr.uky.edu/cis/cis.html; 1-800-422-6237

Cancer support groups: www.supportworks.org

Email: cancernet@icic.nci.nih.gov

Gynecologic Oncology Group: www.gog.org

National Cancer Institute: www.cancernet.nci.nih.gov

National Cervical Cancer Public Education Campaign (American Medical Women's Association): www.cervicalcancer campaign.org

National Coalition for Cancer Survivorship: www.access.digex.net/~mkragen/index. html; 1-301-650-8868

Oncolink: www.oncolink.upenn.edu/

Women's Medical Health Page: www.best.com/~sirlou/whhp.html

Selected References

CHAPTER 1: "CERVICAL CANCER AND HUMAN PAPILLOMAVIRUSES: SEXUALLY TRANSMITTED DISEASES"

American Cancer Society. 2001. *Cancer Facts and Figures.* Atlanta: American Cancer Society.

Aurelian, L., J. D. Strandberg, L. V. Melendez, and L. A. Johnson. 1971. "Herpesvirus Type 2 Isolated from Cervical Tumor Cells Grown in Culture." *Science* 174: 704–707.

Brinton, L. A., R. F. Hamman, G. R. Huggins, H. F. Lehman, R. S. Levine, K. Mallin, and J. F. Fraumeni. 1987. "Sexual and Reproductive Risk Factors for Invasive Squamous Cell Cervical Cancer." *Journal of the National Cancer Institute* 79: 23–30.

Colgan, T. J., R. M. A. Austin, and D. D. Davey. 2001. "The Annual Papanicolaou Test: Women's Safety and Public Policy." *Cancer Cytopathology* 93: 81–85.

Crum, C. P., E. S. Cibas, and K. R. Lee. 1997. *Pathology of Early Cervical Neoplasia.* New York: Churchill Livingston Inc.

Derksen, D. J., and A. Y. Smith. 1989. "Genitourinary Problems in the Male Patient: Benign Conditions of the External Genitalia." *Primary Care* 16: 981–95.

Griffiths, M. 1991. " 'Nuns, Virgins, and Spinsters': Rigoni-Stern and Cervical Cancer Revisited." *British Journal of Obstetrics and Gynecology* 98: 797–802.

Groopman, J. 1999. "Contagion." *New Yorker*, 13 September, pp. 34–49.

Ho, G. Y. F., R. Bierman, L. Beardsley, C. J. Chang, and R. D. Burk. 1998. "Natural History of Cervicovaginal Papillomavirus Infection in Young Women." *New England Journal of Medicine* 338: 423–28.

Janerich, D. T., O. Hadjimichael, P. E. Schwartz, D. M. Lowell, J. W. Meigs, M. J. Merino, J. T. Flannery, and A. P. Polednak. 1995. "The Screening Histories of Women with Invasive Cervical Cancer, Connecticut." *American Journal of Public Health* 85: 791–94.

Kessler, I. I. 1977. "Venereal Factors in Human Cervical Cancer." *Cancer* 39: 1912–19.

Koutsky, L. A., K. K. Holmes, C. W. Critchlow, C. E. Steven, J. Paavonen, A. M. Beckmann, T. A. DeRouen, D. A. Galloway, D. Vernon, and N. B. Kiviat. 1992. "A Cohort Study of Risk of Cervical Intraepithelial Neoplasia Grade 2 or 3 in Relation to Papillomavirus Infection." *New England Journal of Medicine* 327: 1272–78.

Levine, R. U., C. P. Crum, E. Herman, D. Silvers, A. Ferenczy, and R. M. Richart. 1984. "Cervical Papillomavirus Infection and Intraepithelial Neoplasia: A Study of Male Sexual Partners." *Obstetrics and Gynecology* 64: 16–20.

Meyer, T., R. Arndt, E. Christophers, E. Beckmann, S. Schroder, L. Gissman, and E. Stockfleth. 1998. "Association of Rare Human Papillomavirus Types with Genital Premalignant and Malignant Lesions." *Journal of Infectious Diseases* 178: 252–55.

Miller, B. A., L. N. Kolonel, L. Bernstein, J. L. Young Jr., G. M. Swanson, D. West, C. R. Key, J. M. Liff, C. S. Glover, and G. A. Alexander, eds. 1996. *Racial/ Ethnic Patterns of Cancer in the United States 1988–1992.* NIH Publication No. 96-4104. Bethesda, Md.: National Cancer Institute.

Mingo, C. 1998. *Barriers to Screening: More Pap Tests than Mammograms.* Albuquerque, N.Mex.: New Mexico Department of Health, Breast and Cervical Cancer Detection and Control Program.

Nahmias, A. J., Z. M. Naib, and W. E. Josey. 1974. "Epidemiological Studies Relating Genital Herpetic Infection to Cervical Carcinoma." *Cancer Research* 34: 1111–17.

Nasiell, K., V. Roger, and M. Nasiell. 1986. "Behavior of Mild Cervical Dysplasia during Long-term Follow-up." *Obstetrics and Gynecology* 67: 665.

Oriel, J. D. 1971. "Natural History of Genital Warts." *British Journal of Venereal Disease* 47: 1–13.

Parkin, D. M., S. L .Whelan, J. Ferlay, L. Raymond, and J. L. Young. 1997. *Cancer Incidence in Five Continents.* Vol. 7, World Health Organization, International Agency for Research on Cancer (IARC) Scientific Publications No. 143. Lyon, France.

Ries, L. A. G., M. P. Eisner, C. L. Kosary, B. F. Hankey, B. A. Miller, L. X. Clegg, and B. K. Edwards, eds. *SEER Cancer Statistics Review, 1973–1997.* NIH Publication No. 00-2789. Bethesda, Md.: National Cancer Institute.

Sand, P. K., L. W. Bowen, S. O. Blischke, and D. R. Ostergard. 1986. "Evaluation of Male Consorts of Women with Genital Human Papillomavirus Infection." *Obstetrics and Gynecology* 68: 679–81.

Walboomers, J. M. M., M. V. Jacobs, M. M. Manos, F. X. Bosch, J. A. Kummer, K. V. Shah, P. J. F Snijders, J. Peto, C. J. L. M. Meijer, and N. Muñoz. 1999. "Human Papillomavirus Is a Necessary Cause of Invasive Cervical Cancer Worldwide." *Journal of Pathology* 189: 12–19.

Zur Hausen, H. 1987. "Papillomaviruses in Human Cancer." *Applied Pathology* 5:19.

CHAPTER 2: "PAP SMEARS 101"

Bogdanich, W. "The Pap Test Misses Much Cervical Cancer Through Labs' Errors." *Wall Street Journal*, November 2, 1987.

Federal Register. 1992. "Rules and Regulations; Clinical Laboratory Information Act (CLIA) 1988." *Cytology Laboratory* 57 (40): 7196–97.

CHAPTER 3: "HOW TO READ YOUR PAP SMEAR REPORT"

Collins, L. C., H. H. Wang, and G. M. Abu-Jawdeh. "Qualifiers of Atypical Squamous Cells of Undetermined Significance Help in Patient Management." *Modern Pathology* 9: 677–81.

Crum, C. P., D. R. Genest, J. F. Krane, C. Hogan, D. Sun, B. Bellerose, E. Kostopoulou, and K. R. Lee. 1999. "Subclassifying Atypical Squamous Cells in Thin-Prep Cervical Cytology Correlates with Detection of High-Risk Human Papillomavirus DNA." *American Journal of Clinical Pathology* 112: 384–90.

Genest, D. R., B. Dean, K. R. Lee, E. Sheets, C. P. Crum, and E. S. Cibas. 1998. "Qualifying the Cytologic Diagnosis of 'Atypical Squamous Cells of Undetermined Significance' Affects the Predictive Value of a Squamous Intraepithelial Lesion on Subsequent Biopsy." *Archives of Pathology and Laboratory Medicine* 122: 338–41.

Kurman, R. J., and D. Solomon. 1994. *The Bethesda System for Reporting Cervical/Vaginal Cytologic Diagnoses.* New York: Springer-Verlag, Inc.

National Cancer Institute Workshop. 1993. "The Bethesda System for Reporting Cervical/Vaginal Cytologic Diagnoses." *Acta Cytologica* 37: 115–24.

CHAPTER 4: "FOLLOW-UP AND TREATMENT OF ABNORMAL PAP SMEARS: WHAT YOU CAN EXPECT"

American College of Obstetricians and Gynecologists. 1993. *Technical Bulletin*, no. 183.

Malone, J. M. 1997. "Colposcopy and Cervical Biopsy." In *Invasive Outpatient Procedures in Reproductive Medicine*, edited by M. I. Evans, M. P. Johnson, and K. S. Moghissi, pp. 119–28. Philadelphia: Lippincott-Raven Publishers.

Richert, R., and T. C. Wright. 1997. "The Loop Electrosurgical Excision Procedure." In *Invasive Outpatient Procedures in Reproductive Medicine*, edited by M. I. Evans, M. P. Johnson, and K. S. Moghissi, pp. 129–41. Philadelphia: Lippincott-Raven Publishers.

Sheets, E. E. 1999. "The Cervix." In *Kistner's Gynecology and Women's Health*, 7th ed., edited by K. J. Ryan, R. S. Berkowitz, R. L. Barbieri, and A. D. Dunaif, pp. 93–120. St. Louis: Mosby, Inc.

CHAPTER 6: "CERVICAL CANCER: DEALING WITH THE DIAGNOSIS"

Agus, D. B., J. C. Vera, and D. W. Golde. 1999. "Stromal Cell Oxidation: A Mechanism by which Tumors Obtain Vitamin C." *Cancer Research* 59: 4555–58.

Averette, H. E., and H. Nguyen. 1995. "Gynecologic Cancer." In *American Cancer Society Textbook of Clinical Oncology*, edited by G. P. Murphy, W. Lawrence, and R. E. Lenhard. Atlanta: American Cancer Society.

Brown, J., T. Byers, K. Thompson, B. Eldridge, C. Doyle, and A. Williams. 2001. "Nutrition During and After Cancer Treatment: A Guide for Informed Choices for Cancer Survivors." *CA A Cancer Journal for Clinicians* 51: 153–87.

Cannistra, S., and J. M. Niloff. 1996. "Cancer of the Uterine Cervix." *New England Journal of Medicine* 334: 1030–38.

Eifel, P. J., J. S. Berek, and J. T. Thigpen. 1997. "Cancer of the Cervix, Vagina, and Vulva." In *Cancer: Principles and Practice of Oncology*, edited by V. T. DeVita, S. Hellman, and S. A. Rosenberg. Philadelphia: Lippincott-Raven Publishers.

Levenback, C., and M. Morris. 2000. "Cervical Cancer." In *MD Anderson Cancer Center and Memorial Sloan-Kettering Cancer Center Handbook of Gynecologic Oncology*, edited by R. R. Barakat, M. W. Bevers, D. M. Gershensom, and W. J. Hoskins. London: Martin Dunitz Ltd.

National Cancer Institute. 1994. "What You Need to Know About Cancer of the Cervix." *National Institutes of Health Publication 95-2047*.

National Institutes of Health Consensus Statement. 1997. "Development Conference Statement on Cervical Cancer." *Gynecology Oncology* 66: 351–61.

Runowicz, C. P., J. A. Petrek, and T. S. Gansler. 1999. *American Cancer Society: Women and Cancer: A Thorough and Comprehensive Resource for Patients and Their Families.* New York: Villard.

Sheets, E. E. 1999. "The Cervix." In *Kistner's Gynecology and Women's Health*, 7th ed., K. J. Ryan, R. S. Berkowitz, R. L. Barbieri, and A. D. Dunaif, pp. 93–120. St. Louis: Mosby, Inc.

CHAPTER 8: "OBTAINING AN OPTIMAL PAP SMEAR RESULT"

Magnusson, P. K. E., P. Lichtenstein, and U. B. Gyllensten. 2000. "Heritability of Cervical Tumors." *International Journal of Cancer* 88: 698–701.

CHAPTER 9: "THE NEW TECHNOLOGIES: A BETTER PAP SMEAR?"

Atypical Squamous Cells of Undetermined Significance/Low Grade Squamous Intraepithelial Lesion Triage Study (ALTS) Group. 2000. "Human Papillomavirus Testing for Triage of Women with Cytologic Evidence of Low-Grade Squamous Intraepithelial Lesions: Baseline Data from a Randomized Trial." *Journal of the National Cancer Institute* 92: 397–402.

Austin, R. M., and I. Ramzy. 1998. "Increased Detection of Epithelial Cell Abnormalities by Liquid-Based Gynecologic Cytology Preparations: A Review of Accumulated Data." *Acta Cytologica* 42: 178–84.

Check, W. 2000. "Opening the Door to HPV Testing." *CAP Today* 14:1–68.

Colgan, T. J., S. F. Patten, and J. S. J. Lee. 1995. "A Clinical Trial of the AutoPap 300 QC System for Quality Control of Cervicovaginal Cytology in the Clinical Laboratory." *Acta Cytologica* 39: 1191–98.

Cuzik, J., E. Beverly, H. Lo, G. Terry, H. Sapper, I. Mielzynska, A. Lorincz, W.-K. Chan, T. Krausz, and P. Soutter. 1999. "HPV Testing in Primary Screening of Older Women." *British Journal of Cancer* 81: 554–58.

Davey, D. D., and C. A. Armenti. 2000. "HPV Primary Screening for Cervical Cancer: More Pain Than Protection." *Diagnostic Cytology* 22: 333–35.

Kinney, W. K., M. M. Manos, L. B. Hurley, and J. E. Ransley. 1998. "Where's the

High-Grade Cervical Neoplasia? The Importance of Minimally Abnormal Papanicolaou Diagnoses." *Obstetrics and Gynecology* 91: 973–76.

Lee, K. R., R. Ashfaq, G. G. Birdsong, M. E. Corkill, K. M. McIntosh, and S. L. Inhorn. 1997. "Comparison of Conventional Papanicolaou Smears and a Fluid-Based, Thin-Layer System for Cervical Cancer Screening." *Obstetrics and Gynecology* 90: 278–84.

Manos, M. M., W. K. Kinney, L. B. Hurley, M. E. Sherman, J. Shieh-Ngai, R. J. Kurman, J. E. Ransley, B. J. Fetterman, J. S. Hartinger, K. M. McIntosh, G. F. Pawlick, and R. A. Hiatt. 1999. "Identifying Women with Cervical Neoplasia. Using Human Papillomavirus DNA Testing for Equivocal Papanicolaou Results." *Journal of the American Medical Association* 281: 1605–10.

Naryshkin, S. "The False-Negative Fraction for Papanicolaou Smears: How Often Are 'Abnormal' Smears Not Detected by a 'Standard' Screening Cytopathologist?" *Archives of Pathology and Laboratory Medicine* 121: 270–72.

Naryshkin, S., and D. D. Davey. 2000. "Incredibly Low False-Negative Proportion: Watch Out!" *Diagnostic Cytopathology* 22: 63–64.

Schiffman, M., R. Herrero, A. Hildesheim, M. E. Sherman, M. Bratti, S. Wacholder, M. Alfaro, M. Hutchinson, J. Morales, M. D. Greenberg, and A. T. Lorincz. 2000. "HPV DNA Testing in Cervical Cancer Screening: Results from Women in a High-Risk Province of Costa Rica." *Journal of the American Medical Association* 283: 87–93.

Sherman, M. E., and D. Kelly. 1992. "High-Grade Squamous Intraepithelial Lesions and Invasive Carcinoma Following the Report of Three Negative Papanicolaou Smears: Screening Failure or Rapid Progression?" *Modern Pathology* 5: 337–42.

Solomon, D., M. Schiffman, and R. Tarone, for the ALTS Group. 2001. "Comparison of Three Management Strategies for Patients with Atypical Squamous Cells of Undetermined Significance: Baseline Results from a Randomized Trial." *Journal of the National Cancer Institute* 93: 293–99.

Wilbur, D. C., M. U. Prey, W. M. Miller, G. F. Pawlick, and T. J. Colgan. 1998. "The AutoPap System for Primary Screening in Cervical Cytology: Comparing the Results of a Prospective, Intended-Use Study with Routine Manual Practice." *Acta Cytologica* 42: 214–20.

Wright, T. C., L. Denny, L. Kuhn, A. Pollack, and A. Lorincz. 2000. "HPV DNA Testing of Self-Collected Vaginal Samples Compared with Cytologic Screening to Detect Cervical Cancer." *Journal of the American Medical Association* 283: 81–86.

CHAPTER 10: "LIFESTYLE AND CERVICAL CANCER PREVENTION"

Brinton, L. A., G. R. Huggins, H. F. Lehman, K. Mallin, D. A. Savitz, E. Trapido, J. Rosenthal, and R. Hoover. 1986. "Long-term Use of Oral Contraceptives and Risk of Invasive Cervical Cancer." *International Journal of Cancer* 38: 339–44.

Brinton, L. A., C. Schairer, W. Haenszel, P. Stolley, H. F. Lehman, R. Levine, and D. A. Savitz. 1986. "Cigarette Smoking and Invasive Cervical Cancer." *Journal of the American Medical Association* 255: 3265–69.

De la Torre, S., and C. Herman. 1999. "A Description of Teenage Girls' Knowledge and Attitudes Towards Pap Smears in New Mexico." *Journal of Investigative Medicine* 47: 9A.

Dell, D. L., H. Chen, F. Ahmad, and D. E. Stewart. 2000. "Knowledge About Human Papillomavirus Among Adolescents." *Obstetrics and Gynecology* 96: 653–56.

Flagg, E. W., R. J. Coates, and R. S. Greenberg. 1995. "Epidemiologic Studies of Antioxidants and Cancer in Humans." *Journal of American College Nutrition* 14: 419–27.

Gamboa-Pinto, A. J., C. L. Rock, M. G. Ferruzzi, A. B. Schowinsky, and S. J. Schwartz. 1998. "Cervical Tissue and Plasma Concentrations of Alpha-Carotene and Beta-Carotene in Women Are Correlated." *Journal of Nutrition* 128: 1933–36.

Herrero, R., N. Potischman, L. A. Brinton, W. C. Reeves, M. M. Brenes, F. Tenorio, R. C. de Britton, and E. Gaitan. 1991. "A Case-Control Study of Nutrient Status and Invasive Cervical Cancer. I. Dietary Indicators." *American Journal of Epidemiology* 134: 1335–46.

Levy, E., and T. Monte. 1997. *The Ten Best Tools to Boost Your Immune System: A Total Health Prescription.* Boston: Houghton Mifflin Co.

Massion, C. T. 2000. "Nutrients and Cervical Cancer Prevention." *Alternative Therapies in Women's Health* 2: 57–64.

Morabia, A., M. Bernstein, S. Heritier, and N. Khatchatrian. 1996. "Breast Cancer and Smoking." *American Journal Epidemiology* 143: 918–28.

Morrison, E. A. B., G. Y. F. Ho, S. H. Vermund, G. L. Goldberg, A. S. Kadish, K. F. Kelley, and R. D. Burk. 1991. "Human Papillomavirus Infection and Other Risk Factors for Cervical Neoplasia: A Case-Control Study." *International Journal of Cancer* 49: 6–13.

Nagata, C., H. S. Shimizu, H. Yoshikawa, K. Noda, S. Nozawa, A. Yajima, S. Sekiya, H. Sugimori, Y. Hirai, K. Kanazawa, M. Sugase, and T. Kawana. 1999. "Serum Carotenoids and Vitamins and Risk of Cervical Dysplasia from a Case-Control Study in Japan." *British Journal of Cancer* 81: 1234–37.

Potischman, N., and L. A. Brinton. 1996. "Nutrition and Cervical Neoplasia." *Cancer Causes and Control* 7: 113–26.

Prokopczyk, B., J. E. Cox, D. Hoffman, and S. E. Waggoner. 1997. "Identification of Tobacco-Specific Carcinogen in the Cervical Mucus of Smokers and Non-smokers." *Journal of the National Cancer Institute* 89: 868–73.

Willett, W. C. 1999. "Goals for Nutrition in the Year 2000." *CA A Cancer Journal for Clinicians* 49: 331–52.

Ylitalo, N., P. Sorensen, A. Josefsson, M. Frisch, P. Sparen, J. Ponten, U. Gyllensten, M. Melbye, and H.-O. Adami. 1999. "Smoking and Oral Contraceptives as Risk Factors for Cervical Carcinoma In-Situ." *International Journal of Cancer* 81: 357–65.

CHAPTER 11: "NEW DIRECTIONS IN CERVICAL CANCER PREVENTION"

Borysiewicz, L. K., A. Fiander, M. Nimako, S. Man, G. W. G. Wilkinson, D. Westmoreland, A. S. Evans, M. Adams, S. N. Stacey, M. E. G. Boursnell, E. Rutherford, J. K. Hickling, and S. C. Inglis. 1996. "A Recombinant Vaccinia Virus Encoding Human Papillomavirus Types 16 and 18, E6 and E7 Proteins as Immunotherapy for Cervical Cancer." *Lancet* 347: 1523–27.

Breitburd, F., and P. Coursaget. 1999. "Human Papillomavirus Vaccines." *Seminars in Cancer Biology* 9: 431–45.

Cohenford, M. A., T. A. Godwin, F. Cahn, P. Bhandare, T. A. Caputo, and B. Rigas. 1997. "Infrared Spectroscopy of Normal and Abnormal Cervical Smears: Evaluation by Principal Component Analysis." *Gynecologic Oncology* 66: 59–65.

Harro, C. D., Y.-Y. S. Pang, R. B. S. Roden, A. Hildesheim, Z. Wang, M. J. Reynolds, T. C. Mast, R. Robinson, B. R. Murphy, R. A. Karron, J. Dillner, J. T. Schiller, and D. R. Lowry. 2001. "Safety and Immunogenicity Trial in Adult Volunteers of a Human Papillomavirus 16 L1 Virus-Like Particle Vaccine." *Journal of the National Cancer Institute* 93: 284–92.

Hines, J. F., S. Ghim, and A. B. Jenson. 1998. "Prospects for Human Papillomavirus Vaccine Development: Emerging HPV Vaccines." *Current Opinions in Obstetrics and Gynecology* 10: 15–19.

Sano, T., T. Oyaama, K. Kashiwabara, T. Fukuda, and T. Nakajima. 1998. "Immunohistochemical Overexpression of p16 Protein Associated with Intact Retinoblastoma Expression in Cervical Cancer and Cervical Intraepithelial Neoplasia." *Pathology International* 48: 580–85.

Wheeler, C. 1997. "Preventive Vaccines for Cervical Cancer." *Salud Pública de México* (Public Health of Mexico) 39: 283–87.

CHAPTER 12: "YOUR TURN: FREQUENTLY ASKED QUESTIONS ABOUT PAP SMEARS"

Anttila, T., P. Saikku, P. Koskela, A. Bloigu, J. Dillner, I. Ikaheimo, E. Jellum, M. Lehtinen, P. Lenner, T. Hakulinen, A. Narvanen, E. Pukkala, S. Thoresen, L. Youngman, and J. Paavonen. 2001. "Serotypes of *Chlamydia trachomatis* and Risk for Development of Cervical Squamous Cell Carcinoma." *Journal of the American Medical Association* 285: 47–51.

Diamant, A. L., M. A. Schuster, K. McGuigan, and J. Lever. 1999. "Lesbians' Sexual History with Men." *Archives of Internal Medicine* 159: 2730–36.

Frisch, M., B. Glimelius, A. J. C. van den Brule, J. Wohlfahrt, C. J. L. M. Meijer, J. M. M. Walboomers, S. Goldman, C. Svensson, H.-O. Adami, and M. Melbye. 1997. "Sexually Transmitted Infection as a Cause of Anal Cancer." *New England Journal of Medicine* 337: 1350–58.

Kundu, A., and A. A. H. Wade. 1995. "Warts in the Oral Cavity." *Genitourinary Medicine* 71:195.

Leigh, I. M., J. A. G. Buchanan, C. A. Harwood, R. Cerio, and A. Storey. "Role of Human Papillomaviruses in Cutaneous and Oral Manifestations of Immunosuppression." *Journal of Acquired Immune Deficiency Syndromes* 21: S49–S57.

Olufemi, O., H. Deneer, and R. Pierson. 2001. "Human Papillomavirus DNA Detection in Sperm Using Polymerase Chain Reaction." *Obstetrics and Gynecology* 97: 357–60.

Palefsky, J. M. 2000. "Anal Squamous Intraepithelial Lesions in Human Immunodeficiency Virus-Positive Men and Women." *Seminars in Oncology* 27: 471–79.

Palefsky, J. M., E. A. Holly, M. L. Ralston, and N. Jay. 1998. "Prevalence and Risk Factors for Human Papillomavirus Infection of the Anal Canal in Human Immunodeficiency Virus (HIV)-Positive and HIV-Negative Homosexual Men." *Journal of Infectious Diseases* 177: 361–67.

Rankow, E. J., and I. Tessaro. 1998. "Cervical Cancer Risk and Papanicolaou Screening in a Sample of Lesbian and Bisexual Women." *Journal of Family Practice* 46: 139–43.

Glossary

Acetic acid. A dilute vinegar solution used during cervical colposcopy. When applied to the cervix, it highlights areas of SIL.

Adenocarcinoma. A tumor of glandular tissue such as the endocervix. This may be an invasive or in-situ tumor.

Adenocarcinoma in-situ (AIS). A high-grade precancer lesion of the endocervical glandular tissue caused by HPV. In-situ refers to confinement of the lesion to the surface lining of the endocervix. Once it has invaded through the lining, it is no longer "in-situ" and is known as "invasive adenocarcinoma."

Adequacy. A statement on a Pap smear report indicating the suitability of a smear for evaluation. The three types of adequacy statements are Satisfactory, Limited, and Unsatisfactory.

AGUS. Atypical glandular cells of undetermined significance. These are changes in glandular cells that are not normal but fall short of a diagnosis of adenocarcinoma.

ASCUS. Atypical squamous cells of undetermined significance. These are changes in cervical squamous cells that are not normal but fall short of a diagnosis of SIL or cancer. Pap smears with ASCUS diagnoses will often qualify the type of atypia thought to be present, that is, whether it is felt to reflect a dysplasia (ASCUS favor SIL or dysplasia) or a reactive process (ASCUS favor reactive).

Atrophy. A thinning of the lining of the cervix and vagina that occurs with age as the result of decreasing levels of estrogen. These changes can also be seen in individual cells. Older women in menopause may demonstrate atrophic changes on their Pap smears.

Bacterial vaginosis. Presence of abnormal bacteria in the vagina and cervix that indicates a change from the normal bacterial mix at those sites. This may produce inflammation on a Pap smear.

Basement membrane. A thin layer of collagen that underlies the surface lining or epithelium of a body site, such as the cervix. An invasive cancer invades or breaks through the basement membrane to involve deeper tissues.

Benign. Not malignant.

Benign cellular changes (BCC). A Pap smear diagnosis that indicates changes resulting from reactive processes such as infections other than HPV or inflammation from some other cause. Hormonal changes can also result in this diagnosis. Changes of dysplasia are not present in a Pap smear with this diagnosis.

Biopsy. A surgical procedure where a small piece of tissue is removed and sent to a pathology laboratory for a diagnosis. This term also refers to the actual piece of tissue removed.

Broom. A plastic device that resembles a small broom used to collect cells for a Pap smear. The broom is inserted into a woman's endocervical canal and rotated to gather cells from the surface of the cervix.

Brush. A small plastic brush used to collect cells for a Pap smear as described above for a broom.

Cancer. A malignant transformation of tissue. This change is the result of accumulated genetic events within cells that enable a cancer to invade and destroy nearby or distant normal tissues.

Candida. The most common form of fungal infection (or yeast) found on Pap smears. The presence of Candida indicates a vaginal or cervical fungal infection.

Carcinoma. A cancer or malignancy of epithelial tissues such as squamous or glandular tissues. This can be either invasive or in-situ.

Cell. The microscopic subcomponents of tissues such as those of your skin or cervix. Cells are made up of a nucleus and surrounding cytoplasm and can only be seen with the aid of a microscope. Specific changes in cervical cells indicate dysplasia or SIL.

Cervix. The firm, muscular structure at the end of the uterus that opens into the upper portion of the vagina. It is the site of precancers and cancers caused by HPV infection.

Chemotherapy. Chemical treatment of cancer, either given intravenously or by pills. Chemotherapy acts in various ways to arrest the growth and spread of cancer.

Chlamydia. A sexually transmitted bacteria (*Chlamydia trachomatis*) that can cause infection of the cervix as well as the other female reproductive organs, such as the uterus, fallopian tubes, and ovaries. It often, but not always, produces an abnormal cervical discharge. If untreated by antibiotics, this infection can cause severe scarring of tissues that can result in infertility.

CIN. Cervical Intraepithelial Neoplasia. An older term which is synonymous with dysplasia, precancer, and SIL.

Clinician. A physician, nurse, nurse practitioner, or physician's assistant who provides medical care.

Colposcopy. A procedure that allows close examination of the cervix using a binoculars-like device for magnification of the surface of the cervix. This is performed in the process of detection, biopsy, and treatment of SILs.

Compromised immune state. Any situation in which the body's normal immune defenses are not fully functional. It is said that people with this problem are immunocompromised. Examples of this are seen during treatment with certain drugs such as those given to organ transplant recipients and cancer patients receiving radiation therapy. Infection by the human immunodeficiency virus (HIV) leading to the Acquired Immunodeficiency Syndrome (AIDS) is another example.

Condyloma. The medical term for genital warts that are fleshy, warty lesions found on the external genital and anal areas of men and women. These are caused by low-risk forms of HPV.

Cone. A surgical procedure that removes a conical portion of the cervix. This is used to treat some HSILs and AIS.

Curettage. A surgical procedure that scrapes the lining of the endocervical canal for diagnostic purposes.

Cystitis. Inflammation of the lining of the bladder that may occur as a result of therapy for cervical cancer.

Cytopathologist. A physician trained in pathology who has additional training in cytopathology, the study of cells for medical diagnoses. Pap smears represent the major type of specimens which cytopathologists examine. Cytopathologists are the ones who make a final diagnosis on abnormal Pap smears.

Cytoplasm. The material that forms the bulk of a cell's volume and surrounds the cell's nucleus.

Cytotechnologist. A medical laboratory technologist whose job it is to examine Pap smears searching for abnormal cells, such as those diagnostic of SIL or dysplasia. Pap smears with abnormal cells found by a cytotechnologist are sent to a cytopathologist for a final diagnosis.

Dysplasia. A cervical precancerous or precursor lesion. This is synonymous with SIL and CIN.

Endocervix. The upper portion of the cervix which is lined by glandular or endocervical cells.

Endometrium. A type of glandular tissue that lines the uterus. This lining is shed each month during a woman's menstrual period.

Epithelium. General term referring to the skin and the lining of body cavities. The cervix is covered by two types of epithelium, squamous and endocervical (or glandular).

External beam. A method of delivering radiation therapy for cervical cancer whereby radiation is directed to the tumor from outside the body.

Fungus. A microorganism that can infect the body. Candida is an example of a common vaginal fungal infection. Fungus is also known as "yeast."

Genital wart. Also known as "condyloma," a fleshy, warty HPV lesion found on the external genital and anal region of men and women.

Glandular. A type of epithelium that has the ability to produce secretions. In the cervix, glandular epithelium covers the endocervix.

Gonorrhea. A sexually transmitted bacterial infection caused by *Neisseria gonorrhoeae*. It may cause an abnormal cervical discharge in women or it may be asymptomatic. Failure to treat this infection with antibiotics can lead to infertility due to involvement and scarring of the fallopian tubes.

Gynecologist. A physician with specialty training in women's health.

Herpes simplex virus. A family of viruses, some of which can be sexually transmitted and cause sores on a woman's or man's genitals. Herpes causes changes in squamous cells that can be detected on a Pap smear. Other types of herpes are not sexually transmitted, for example, the type that causes cold sores around the mouth.

High-grade squamous intraepithelial lesion (HSIL). A cervical precancer lesion that has a high risk of progressing to cervical cancer if untreated. This type of SIL is typically caused by high-risk HPV types such as HPV 16 and 18.

Human papillomavirus (HPV). A large family of viruses which cause warts as well as cancerous and precancerous changes in various tissues of the male and female reproductive tract. HPV is known to be the causative agent of cervical and penile cancers.

Hysterectomy. A surgical procedure that removes a woman's uterus. The cervix is usually removed with the uterus during this operation. This may be performed as treatment for cancer or more commonly for nonmalignant reasons.

Inflammation. The process whereby white blood cells accumulate. This may be to fight infection or for some other biologic reason.

In-situ. A characteristic of malignancies whereby they are confined to the lining where they originate. This is in contrast to invasive tumors that are not confined and have the ability to invade surrounding tissues and possibly metastasize to distant sites.

Intracavitary radiation. A form of radiation therapy for cervical cancer whereby a radioactive cylinder is placed inside a woman's vagina. The cylinder delivers radioactivity directly (transvaginally) to the cervical cancer that serves to shrink the tumor.

Invasive. A characteristic of tumors that reflects their ability to invade surrounding tissues.

Lesion. A growth of tissue. May produce a lump, irregularity, or discoloration in the tissue or it may be invisible to the naked eye.

Lidocaine. A local anesthetic, identical to xylocaine® used in dental procedures, used during surgical procedures on the cervix, such as a loop. Lidocaine is injected into the cervix to temporarily numb the area prior to the procedure.

Limited. A statement of adequacy on a Pap smear report that indicates that the Pap smear was less than optimal for evaluation and diagnosis.

Liquid-based Pap smear. A modification of the traditional Pap smear where cells are immediately placed into a liquid preservative instead of smeared on a glass slide.

Loop. A surgical procedure that employs hot electrocautery tools to remove tissue from the cervix. This is also commonly referred to as Loop Electrocautery Excision Procedure or LEEP®.

Low-grade squamous intraepithelial lesion (LSIL). A cervical precancer lesion showing changes resulting from infection by HPV. This lesion has a low risk of progressing to cervical cancer. This type of SIL is typically caused by low-risk HPV types such as HPV 6 and 11.

Lugol's solution. A yellow iodine-based solution used during colposcopy to highlight areas of the cervix suspicious for dysplasia. A clinician can then biopsy any areas of concern.

Malignant. The property of a cancer that allows it to invade and destroy normal tissues.

Menopause. The time in a woman's life when her menstrual periods have ceased.

Metastasis. The spread of an invasive tumor to lymph nodes or distant sites. This can happen either through blood or lymph vessels.

Monsel's paste. A dark iron-containing paste used during cervical biopsies and loops to stop bleeding. The paste is applied directly to the bleeding site.

Negative. A term used in medicine to mean a test such as a Pap smear is normal.

Neoplasia. A general term for a tumor (a neoplasm), which is a change in tissues demonstrating abnormal or uncontrolled growth. This can be either benign or malignant.

Normal. A Pap test diagnosis that indicates there is no evidence of abnormal or atypical cells on the smear. This diagnosis is often phrased as "within normal limits" or "negative."

Nucleus. The structure within a cell that contains the cell's genetic material or DNA. Abnormal changes in the appearance of a cell's nucleus are characteristic of SILs and cancer.

Oncologist. A physician with specialty training in the treatment of cancers. A gynecologic oncologist is a physician who specifically treats women with malignancies of their reproductive or female organs.

Papanicolaou. Dr. George Papanicolaou (1883–1962), the originator of the Pap smear, developed it from 1920–1940. It was during this time that it was introduced as a screening test for cervical cancer in the United States.

Pap smear. A screening test for cervical cancer that removes cells from a woman's cervix and places them on a slide for examination by a microscope. This test can also detect precancerous changes in cells.

Pathologist. A physician with a specialty in pathology, the study of diseases of the human body. Using a microscope, a pathologist makes diagnoses on specimens taken from patients such as Pap smears and cervical biopsies, among many others.

Perimenopause. The time in a woman's life when she is approaching menopause or the cessation of her menstrual periods. Although perimenopausal women will still have menstrual periods, their periods may be irregular and unusual in timing, length, and heaviness.

Positive. A term used in medicine to indicate that a test has abnormal results.

Postmenopause. The time in a woman's life when she has ceased having menstrual periods.

Precancer. A change in tissues that falls short of a diagnosis of cancer. In the cervix, these changes indicate the presence of HPV.

Radiation therapy. A form of cancer therapy, used frequently in treating cervical cancer. A dose of radiation is directed to the tumor that acts to shrink the tumor. Radiation for cervical cancer can be given from outside the body (external beam) or from inside using radioactive implants in the vagina (intracavitary radiation).

Report. The form generated by a cytology laboratory that gives your Pap smear diagnosis.

Requisition. The form that accompanies a Pap smear from the clinic or doctor's office where the smear was taken. This form contains a woman's important personal information such as her name, date of birth, last menstrual period, date the Pap smear was collected, and pertinent medical history.

Satisfactory. The designation of Pap smear adequacy that indicates a Pap smear is of sufficient quality for examination and diagnosis.

Screen. The initial examination of a Pap smear performed by cytotechnologists whereby a Pap smear is viewed using a microscope with the goal of detecting abnormalities in cells. If no abnormalities are seen, the cytotechnologist reports the Pap smear as "normal" or "negative."

Sexually transmitted diseases (STD). Also known as sexually transmitted infections (STI), these represent a variety of diseases that are passed between sexual partners during sex. Common sexually transmitted diseases include HPV, herpes, trichomonas, chlamydia, gonorrhea, and syphilis.

Slide. A thin piece of glass, about the size of a stick of gum. The cells collected from the cervix for a Pap smear are placed on the slide. After staining, the slide is examined under a microscope for abnormalities.

Spatula. A wooden device used for collecting cells from the cervix for a Pap smear. It is placed in the cervical opening and rotated around gathering cells from the surface.

Squamous. The type of epithelial lining which covers the outer portion of the cervix and the vagina.

Stage. A term indicating the extent of spread of a cancer. Cervical cancers are given a stage between I-IV with Stage I being the least advanced.

Stain. A set of solutions used to color cells or tissues so they are visible when examined by a microscope. The stain used for Pap smears is called the "Papanicolaou stain."

Stenosis. A narrowing of an opening such as the endocervical canal in cervical stenosis. Cervical stenosis may occur naturally in women as they age. It can also occur as a consequence of surgical therapy for dysplasia.

Subtypes. The number by which the various members of the HPV family are designated. Common sexually transmitted HPV subtypes in this country include HPV 6, 11, 16, 18, and 31.

Syphilis. A sexually transmitted bacterial infection caused by *Treponema pallidum*. This infection results in the formation of chancres, which are solitary painless ulcerations occurring at the site of infection. If untreated by antibiotics, syphilis can develop into a long-term infection involving other parts of the body.

Thin-layer Pap smear. Another name for liquid-based Pap smears, a modification of the traditional Pap smear.

Transformation zone. The area of the cervix where the squamous lining meets the endocervical or glandular lining. This is also the site of HPV infection and where most cervical SILs arise. Also known as the "transition zone."

Transvaginal radiation. See **intracavitary radiation**.

Trichomonas. Also known as "Trich," the sexually transmitted parasite *Trichomonas vaginalis* that can produce reactive or inflammatory changes on a Pap smear.

Tumor. An abnormal growth of tissue. A tumor may be benign or malignant.

Unsatisfactory. The designation of adequacy on a Pap smear that indicates that a Pap smear is of too inferior quality for examination and diagnosis. No diagnosis will be given and the Pap smear should be repeated.

Vaginal intraepithelial lesion (VAIN). A dysplasia or precancer located in the vagina that reflects infection by HPV at that site. VAINs can be either low or high grade which, as with cervical SILs, have either a low or high risk of progressing to cancer.

Vulvar intraepithelial lesion (VIN). A dysplasia or precancer located on the vulva that reflects an infection by HPV at that site. VINs can be either low or high grade which, as with cervical SILs, have either a low or high risk of progressing to cancer.

Within normal limits. A Pap smear diagnosis, which states that no abnormalities are detected. Also known as a "negative" Pap smear.

Yeast. A term that is used interchangeably with "fungus" in the vagina. A common fungal infection of the vagina and cervix caused is by *Candida albicans*. This infection may produce inflammation on a Pap smear.

Index

265